THE AUTISM DIALOGUE APPROACH HANDBOOK

The Autism Dialogue Approach Handbook serves as both a comprehensive guide and a practical handbook for healthcare professionals, educators, caregivers and anyone engaging with the autism community. Jonathan Drury presents the Autism Dialogue Approach (ADA), a pioneering framework rooted in dialogue and mindfulness practices. It addresses the diverse needs of autistic and neurodivergent individuals, emphasising that 'the autism community' includes everyone, promoting an inclusive understanding of neurodiversity.

The book critiques traditional therapeutic and coaching models, proposing ADA as an alternative that values co-creation and shared meaning-making. By exploring practical strategies, Drury demonstrates how ADA transforms therapy, coaching and leadership by fostering environments where neurodivergent and neurotypical individuals can connect authentically and transcend division. With clear tools, exercises and real-world examples, this handbook guides readers in applying ADA to cultivate neurodivergent-affirming, inclusive spaces. It also delves into the philosophical and spiritual dimensions of dialogue, offering insights into how societal structures impact autistic experiences and how systemic change can occur through dialogue.

Aimed at those committed to building compassionate and inclusive settings, this handbook equips readers with practical skills for nurturing deep connections, promoting wellbeing and driving societal transformation through a neurodiversity-affirming approach.

Jonathan Drury has been an expert in autism, neurodiversity and environmental trauma for over ten years, working with individuals, teams and organisations across the UK and internationally. He has designed experiential programmes that explore the healing power of dialogue from a unique and universal perspective, and a range of transformative tools and approaches for wider perspectives and deeper understanding in autism wellbeing and leadership. His work has empowered countless individuals to navigate their lives with increased confidence and clarity. A regular speaker and trainer, Jonathan draws on ancient health philosophies, somatic awareness, the arts, spiritual disciplines and many established dialogue modalities to offer a fresh lens on neurodiversity and leadership. *The Autism Dialogue Approach Handbook* is his first book.

'The Autism Dialogue provides an insightful perspective… [and] aims to replace a negative deficit-based view with teaching people about the benefits of autistic ways of perceiving the world.'

Temple Grandin, *author of* Visual Thinking and Thinking in Pictures, *USA*

'This text succinctly outlines the value of the Autism Dialogue Approach and the ways it can be used to enable deeper communication, respect and connection.'

Professor Elizabeth Milne, *Professor of Cognitive Neuroscience, The University of Sheffield, UK*

'a vital contribution to researchers and practitioners across many fields.'

Lori Hogenkamp, *Center for Adaptive Stress, USA*

'With this impressive handbook, Jonathan not only emancipates "Autism" from the shackles of conventional labelling, he also provides us all – whatever our neurotype – with deeply considered ideas to help us fully embrace our own uniqueness and that of others.'

Vincent Traynor, *Associate Professor of Change Leadership, Sheffield Business School*

'With this book, Jonathan offers us the gift of a veritable view from within the world of autistic experience, a perspective that takes seriously the notion that practical knowledge about human experience is the royal road – and the active principle – for understanding how our minds are not isolated but work together to bring forth meaningful worlds.'

Amy Cohen Varela, *Clinical Psychologist, Chair of Mind & Life Europe, Switzerland*

'The principles of Autism Dialogue are eloquently explained in this innovative book. It provides the reader with insights into a strengths-based approach that can empower. The author invites us to consider the richness of lived experiences via self and mutual understanding. This approach has great potential to reduce harmful societal misunderstandings of autism. The Autism Dialogue Approach needs to be embraced.'

Megan Freeth, *Professor of Neurodevelopmental Psychology. University of Sheffield, UK*

The Autism Dialogue Approach Handbook

Transforming Communication in Neurodiversity

Jonathan Drury

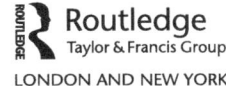

LONDON AND NEW YORK

Cover image credit: Jonathan Drury

First published 2025
by Routledge
4 Park Square, Milton Park, Abingdon, Oxon OX14 4RN

and by Routledge
605 Third Avenue, New York, NY 10158

Routledge is an imprint of the Taylor & Francis Group, an informa business

© 2025 Jonathan Drury

The right of Jonathan Drury to be identified as author of this work has been asserted in accordance with sections 77 and 78 of the Copyright, Designs and Patents Act 1988.

All rights reserved. No part of this book may be reprinted or reproduced or utilised in any form or by any electronic, mechanical, or other means, now known or hereafter invented, including photocopying and recording, or in any information storage or retrieval system, without permission in writing from the publishers.

Trademark notice: Product or corporate names may be trademarks or registered trademarks, and are used only for identification and explanation without intent to infringe.

British Library Cataloguing-in-Publication Data
A catalogue record for this book is available from the British Library

Library of Congress Cataloging-in-Publication Data
Names: Drury, Jonathan, author.
Title: The autism dialogue approach handbook : transforming communication in neurodiversity / Jonathan Drury.
Description: Abingdon, Oxon ; New York, NY : Routledge, 2025. | Includes bibliographical references and index.
Identifiers: LCCN 2024049864 (print) | LCCN 2024049865 (ebook) | ISBN 9781032668086 (hardback) | ISBN 9781032668079 (paperback) | ISBN 9781032668116 (ebook)
Subjects: LCSH: Autistic people--Social conditions. | Autistic people--Psychology. | Interpersonal communication.
Classification: LCC HV1570.23 .D78 2025 (print) | LCC HV1570.23 (ebook) | DDC 616.85/8820014--dc23/eng/20250130
LC record available at https://lccn.loc.gov/2024049864
LC ebook record available at https://lccn.loc.gov/2024049865

ISBN: 978-1-032-66808-6 (hbk)
ISBN: 978-1-032-66807-9 (pbk)
ISBN: 978-1-032-66811-6 (ebk)

DOI: 10.4324/9781032668116

Typeset in Sabon LT Pro
by KnowledgeWorks Global Ltd.

*To Paul
and the Eternal Dialogue*

Contents

Foreword by Kate Salinsky — xi
Preface — xiii
Acknowledgements — xvi

PART I WHAT ARE WE DEALING WITH HERE? 1

1 What brings us here? 3
Growing up — 4
The seeds of Autism Dialogue — 5
First experiments with dialogue — 8
A handbook — 10
How to read this book — 11

2 Autism as a way of being 13
Discovery journey — 13
Autistic culture — 18

3 Dialogue in historical context 20
Traditional communities and societies — 21
Dialogue and indigenous societies — 22
East and west dialogues — 24
Dialogue in practice — 25

4 Bringing together autism and Dialogue 28
The importance of mindful awareness — 31
Experiences in early Dialogue sessions — 32

PART II COMMUNITIES OF MEANING-MAKING — 37

5 Introduction to Dialogue in autism contexts — 39
- The key principles and aims of Autism Dialogue — 39
- Explicit aims — 40
- The four practices — 41
- Using the four practices in a group — 42
- Further considerations around sensitive conversation — 43
- The benefits of an ADA practice — 45

6 Autism theories and common themes — 47
- What is autism? — 48
- Autism as a way of being — 49
- Monotropism — 50
- Stress adaptation — 51
- Double empathy — 52
- Autistic communication styles — 53
- Autistic peer-to-peer information transfer is highly effective — 53
- Sensory sensitivity: the intense world — 54
- Masking — 54
- Trauma – an introduction — 55
- Other problems that autistic individuals may face — 56
- The need for dialogues in autism — 56

7 Autism and Dialogue through the lens of social sciences — 59
- Nature of self — 61
- Dialogue as a system — 62
- Letting be, thinking, participatory sense-making and generative dialogue — 63
- Bohm's theory of Wholeness and the Implicate Order — 64
- Systemic trauma — 65
- Lockdown — 67
- How can Dialogue address communication breakdown? — 68

8 Neurodiversity — 71
- Neurodiversity paradigm and intersectionality, in a Yorkshire accent — 72
- Problems with neurodiversity — 72
- Does the neurodiversity paradigm compare to autistic gestalt processing? — 73
- So do we need neurodiversity and, if so, why? — 74

9 Autism Dialogue and mindfulness — 76
- Introduction to mindfulness — 77
- Silence — 78
- Mindful talking and awareness in dialogue groups — 79
- Some thoughts on self-acceptance — 80

	Interoception	81
	Effortless effort	81
	Mantras, moving and other creative devices	82
	Some evidence	83

10 Guide to hosting an Autism Dialogue — 85

- Introduction — 85
- How to prepare for a Dialogue — 86
- Let's begin! — 88
- When boundaries aren't in place — 93
- Closure — 94
- Recording feedback — 94

11 Autism Dialogue facilitation skills — 96

- Participatory considerations — 97
- Digital age — 97
- Facilitating dialogue: responsibility and ethics — 98
- Ethical considerations — 99
- Evaluating dialogue: the art of not knowing and navigating uncertainty — 99
- Facilitating the generative potential of dialogue — 100
- The Autism Dialogue Approach: training for facilitators — 101
- Qualities of an ADA-trained practitioner — 101
- Autistic-only group? — 102
- Working with an organisation — 102
- Professional Dialogue — 104

PART III WIDER CONTEXTS — 107

12 Intersectionality and Dialogue — 109

- Intergroup Dialogue — 111
- The Cycles of Socialisation and Liberation — 113

13 Insight Dialogue and other models — 116

- Pedagogy of the Oppressed — 118
- Dialogism and ethical and spiritual interaction: Bohm, Buber and Bakhtin — 119
- Circles of Trust — 121
- The Socratic Seminar — 121
- World Café — 122

14 Autism Dialogue in therapy and coaching — 123

- Autism and existence — 124
- Talking — 125
- An enactive approach to the helping relationship — 125

Autistic trauma   128
  Masking and the therapeutic process: the role of interaction   128
  Dialogic supervision   129
  The importance of safe, neurodivergent-affirming therapeutic spaces   129
  Relational humility and the paradigm shift in therapy   130
  Training and implementation: ADA as a transformative practice   131
  Conclusion: towards a more inclusive and relationally engaged
     therapeutic practice   131

15 Spirituality in Autism Dialogue   134
  Non-Violent Communication   135
  Spiritual community   135
  Spiritual practice and the inner world of autistic people   136

16 Resistance to change   140
  An autistic leadership culture   141

Appendix 1
Case example: Autism Dialogue in Derby City and Derbyshire
(England, UK)   143

Appendix 2
Case example: community online series 2022   148

Appendix 3
Case example: post-dialogue group community – 'Autism
Dialogue friends'   153

Appendix 4
Case example: Autism Dialogue coaching   155

Appendix 5
Case example: an encounter   160

Appendix 6
A note on research and evaluation   163

Appendix 7
An open letter about communication   166

Index   170

Foreword

I have been a trainer, facilitator and mentor for over 25 years now working in the voluntary and community sector for a long time in substance use and mental health. I began to pursue an interest in neurodivergence initially training as a specialist literacy teacher for dyslexia and moved into working one-to-one with neurodivergent students in higher education in 2014. I first met Jonathan in 2019 when he was studying for a postgraduate diploma in coaching and I was an academic learning adviser at Sheffield Hallam University – a role I still hold, among others. Jonathan sought my advice on one of his academic assignments and I remember Jonathan's passion for his topic and his thoughtful and insightful observations. We explored some ideas for structure and the process of writing an assignment together and he went on his way.

After my child received an autism diagnosis I embarked on a Masters in Autism at Sheffield Hallam University. I wanted to further my understanding so that I might be a better parent and advocate for my autistic child, as well as support my neurodivergent students as best I could. As part of my desire to learn about autism from autistic people, I signed up for an online series of autism dialogue sessions that had been flagged up to students on the MA course as potentially of interest. When I turned up, I realised that the facilitator was Jonathan – the same student whose ideas had intrigued me so much earlier that same year and he immediately recognised me too. This series of online dialogues was unlike any other group (online or otherwise) I had ever experienced. The pace of interaction was slowed and felt deliciously unhurried. I learned to listen to myself and others with a new curiosity and suspension of judgement. I experienced a feeling of collective sense-making as well as personal insights and understandings and always left feeling replenished. Afterwards, standard interactions such as work meetings felt incredibly inferior by comparison – I became aware of how much communication is by monologue or debate, and I had the appetite for more autism dialogue in my life.

As fortune would have it, at the end of the series Jonathan invited me to join him by becoming a director of the recently formed company Dialogic Action and I accepted without hesitation. Since then, Jonathan and I, with the support of our colleagues at Dialogica, have run many more autism dialogues, worked with communities and organisations and developed training for therapists in the Autism Dialogue Approach (ADA). We have also had the opportunity to work together with the Anna Freud Centre and AT-Autism on the National Autism Trainer Programme (NATP) since 2023. As well as colleagues we have become firm friends.

It has been a joy and a privilege to have co-facilitated alongside Jonathan – there have been a few hair-raising moments too, I'm not going to lie! But Jonathan has such intuition and wisdom as a facilitator and has created an approach that really works for bringing neurotypes together; I have always felt safe and supported by him. I wish I had been able to read this book at the start of my journey as an Autism Dialogue practitioner. It is the culmination of many years of Jonathan's work, and it successfully presents a guide to this unique approach which has many philosophical strands (some of which could be quite hard to get to grips with, yet Jonathan has managed to make them accessible). There are also some easily learned practices that you can start using straight away. Having read the book, I have a much better understanding of some of the things Jonathan has been trying to teach me over the years!

One of the things that drew me in to autism dialogue is how it brings together people from different neurotypes and creates a micro-community wherein the dominant deficit neuro-majority narratives are discarded, and the participants create an equitable community in which all are welcome and valued, respected, trusted, listened to and heard. Autism Dialogue creates acceptance, belonging and connection in ways I have not experienced anywhere else. The principles and practices can be applied in all contexts where we interact and relate to others – in therapy and helping relationships, in personal and family relationships and in work contexts too. Jonathan also taught me that the people who show up to dialogue are the right people and that right action follows right thinking. Since you've shown up and are reading this, I trust that you too will take what you need from this book, and I know that ADA can transform your practice and your relationships too – so trust in the process and enjoy the ride.

Kate Salinsky

Preface

Picture a time you were somewhere with friends or family, perhaps in a cosy living room, laughter in the air as you swap stories, jokes, and memories, the atmosphere brimming with a feeling of genuine connection; a poignant reminder of the incomparable happiness found in human interaction. There's an enchanting simplicity in the act of gathering, whether it's enjoying a relaxed meal with loved ones, sitting around a crackling bonfire under a starlit sky, at a spiritual gathering, or merely sharing comfortable silence side by side. In these moments, grand plans, extravagant ambitions and even the sense of being an individual fades into insignificance; a true delight emerges naturally from the simple act of being present with one another.

However, in our rapidly moving world, these instances and opportunities for them can easily slip past unnoticed. We're perpetually bombarded with distractions vying for our attention, dragging us away from the people and moments that hold deeper significance. We've grown accustomed to communicating through texts, emojis, and virtual interactions, for expressing our opinions and positions. There's a constant hum of notifications and the relentless pressure to consistently perform and outdo. Despite being more digitally interconnected than ever, we often feel detached and solitary. In an age dominated by productivity and competing ideologies, the true essence of togetherness has become somewhat obscured.

> Communication breakdown, it's always the same
> Havin' a nervous breakdown, a-drive me insane
>
> (Led Zeppelin, 1969)

Amid the whirlwind of contemporary existence, there exists a yearning for something deeper, something more profound. It's an ache for genuine human interaction, for the type of camaraderie that blossoms from shared encounters and mutual experiences. It's an acknowledgement that, despite our disparities, we are all united by an inherent craving for companionship and acceptance. In the distinct richness that comes from face-to-face encounters, that's where dialogue happens.

I'm an artist really. I didn't think I was a writer, but creativity flows all around us, in us and through us. We're swirled around and swept along as meaning takes shape then slips away. We are all made out of stuff and wordstuff. My art is dialogue. Thinking and languaging became the tools of my craft on a fine art degree, which facilitated the birth of this book, this word, this meaning, this painting, this tune, this pattern, this poem, this prayer, this child …

Looking back, I see that my lifelong journey of self-enquiry began at the age of five, when I experienced a moment of profound insight, realising that the world my elders presented was not the whole picture. I sensed something else lay behind that which was being presented; a hidden order. This led to a quest for deeper understanding that spanned my childhood then adolescence and beyond, with the exploration of altered states of consciousness through psychotropic plants, gnostic self-study and silent retreats. These experiences eventually culminated in the creation of the book you're reading now. I'm hesitant to apologise for the amount of subjective experience I bring into this book, so I won't.

Being open to life, to unlearning and unknowing means we can taste and be more aligned with the flow of life and meaning-making, with a childlike curiosity. Being a dialogue facilitator means I continue to learn experientially, to forget myself, my identities, categories, titles and fixedness of thought, which means being open to outside influences of all types. I exercised my authentic voice in Sufi community gatherings for over 20 years. Like many others, I repeatedly found myself with eyes closed and mouth open to let the heart speak its supplication and reflection. In front of many people, the ritual gathering allows the heart to be heard by others with respect and without judgement, as if speaker, listener and message are one unified whole. When storytelling too, at pub events and workshops, the power of being unified with a group of listeners is incredible, as the audience seems somehow to draw the telling out of the teller. My kids were my best audience by far, and that's another true story.

My journey with Autism Dialogue began in 2014 after I was informed I met the criteria for Asperger Syndrome, which I didn't believe, but then I've always wondered what 'belief' and 'knowing' really mean too! I wonder and my words wander. Notably, the word diagnosis was never used, but feeling the need to take advantage of various support mechanisms in university and at work, I found the word is widely used in autism. In turn, this realisation led to me wanting to dismantle the word; *dia* means through or between (it's the same in *dialogue*) and *gnosis* means knowing. The word isn't medical at all so you don't have to say you were 'diagnosed with autism' if no one's told you that you were. Language holds power and I think this realisation is where my Autism Dialogue journey really started.

I attended talking support groups and while these sessions offered some consolation, I felt they didn't offer what was possible. I'd just come out of 20 years of societal exile in a Turkish Sufi order and another three years of silent retreats and studying Advaita and Vipassana. As someone with a degree in Contemporary Fine Art and years of experience organising arts events and in deeply creative and spiritual communities, I was drawn to the idea of creating something deeper, more embodied and more expansive. I recalled my previous work with Bohm Dialogue, since uni, which became the foundation for what would later evolve into Autism Dialogue.

REFERENCE

Led Zeppelin (1969). Communication Breakdown [song] On *Led Zeppelin*. Atlantic Records.

Acknowledgements

I wish to thank the many people who have helped make this book a reality.

Heartfelt gratitude goes to Professor Liz Milne at the University of Sheffield for the spark which lit that first Autism Dialogue, and her ensuing years of encouragement and Dr Richard Smith at SAANS who suggested I contact Liz about my autism dialogue idea in the first place. A bow of gratitude also goes to Hester Reeve and Helen Blejerman for bringing Dialogue into the Fine Art curriculum at Hallam when I was there. All of the above was such excellent timing!

Special thanks to Kate Salinsky for bringing her incredible training experience into the dialogue arena, and for years of patience with my organic style. I've watched Kate become an outstanding facilitator over the years.

Deepest thanks to Dr Hanne De Jaegher for the friendship, conversation and sincere dedication to the great work that always shines through, and extra praise for arranging my visit to UBC to co-facilitate with me the Autism Dialogue session 'Reframing dialogue through embodied approaches: surpassing barriers to health in a verbal world'.

Thank you to Jackie Elliott for friendship, grounding, warmth and our endless hours of co-coaching. Thank you Jane Ball and Peter Garrett at the Academy of Professional Dialogue for early mentoring and helping me become a professional, and for permission to reproduce our work 'Autism Dialogue in Derby City and Derbyshire'.

Sparkling thanks to my great friend Mick Beck for listening and laughs; Nicola Phillips for quality thinking time and whose books are as inspiring and up front as she is; Ahmed Ridwan Burgess for our many quality dialogues over coffee, and Wendy-Ann Fishwick for her introduction to Grace McInnes at Routledge.

Thanks to Nick, Helen, Holly, Hanne and Jackie for direction at the social enterprise stage, to all co-facilitators and all the willing people who have gathered at Autism Dialogue sessions since 2017 who have been at the heart of its success. I feel genuine fellowship with you all.

Thank you to all our funders and clients and many colleagues at organisations especially UHRI, AT-Autism, Anna Freud Centre, Scottish Autism, Sheffield Quaker Centre, Sheffield Hallam Autism and Coaching tutors, all my incredible book endorsers. So sorry if I've forgotten anyone, I am eternally grateful to you all for believing.

Thank you to my beautiful kids for tolerating my absence, and for always reminding me of life and love beyond definition.

And to Katie, my beautiful wife and partner for endless, inspiring conversations, patience, support and unbelievable last-minute editing skills.

PART I

What are we dealing with here?

CHAPTER 1

What brings us here?

In today's fast-paced world, we rarely have the opportunity to sit together in a group setting without the pressure to conform, perform, or deliver a particular outcome. Whatever our neurotype, our society often lacks the time and space for genuine connection and mutual understanding. However, there is a way to bridge this gap: through the practice of Dialogue, a specific method that fosters slow-paced, structured conversation. In Dialogue, we are given a confidential and safe space to unfold ourselves, to learn from each other, to gain new insights, and to feel more empowered in our understanding of ourselves and the world.

When we bring the subject of autism into dialogue, it transforms from a label into a fertile ground for self-enquiry. It becomes a question rather than a definitive category – an open space for exploring what it means to be oneself in a world that often misunderstands or marginalises differences. The Autism Dialogue Approach, therefore, is not merely about understanding autism; it is about exploring the nature of selfhood itself. It challenges the reductionist view that a self can be 'deficient' or 'damaged' and instead, embraces the complexity and richness of autistic experiences as a pathway to greater self-awareness and mutual understanding.

The Autism Dialogue Approach is influenced by many questions and disciplines, from the mysteries of eastern and western philosophy, social cognitive science and definitions of selfhood, to the pathologising tendencies and fragmented mentalities that often characterise discussions around autism. It seeks to dismantle the dichotomy between autistic and non-autistic, or neurodivergent and neurotypical, recognising instead the shared sensitivity to fragmented systems and the common experience of marginalisation. It might be described as a new form of psycho-social coaching, fostering recovery, insight and understanding for all participants, whether autistic or simply different. But different to what?

Many participants in my dialogues have shared that the experience increased their familiarity, self-awareness and compassion for others, reduced their anxiety and stress, and brought new meaning to their lives. By listening to and learning from the experiences of autistic individuals, in structured conversations, we can alleviate the negative impacts of societal misunderstanding and create a more inclusive and supportive environment. The stories of autistic people, expressed through ancient cave art, outstanding inventions, contemporary media and internet writings and activism, offer invaluable insights that challenge reductive scientific approaches and point towards a more humane and empathetic understanding of neurodiversity, that subset of biodiversity and a word that has become another crystallised social construct. In our Dialogues we pause, hold our words up to the light, etymologically dissect them and feel our way into their energies.

Autism, in this context, is not a deficit but an opportunity – a mirror that reflects our own societal shortcomings and calls us to deeper engagement with ourselves and each other. The Autism Dialogue Approach provides a space for sustained collective enquiry, addressing the crisis of communication and the loss of selfhood that affects us all. Through years of practice and participant feedback, it has become clear that it fosters wellbeing and empowerment for autistic individuals and their families, helping to create a more inclusive and dynamic world.

GROWING UP

At several different schools on 13 occasions grown adults struck my hand with a cane, including once for escaping the grounds and running home to avoid the class bully. Psychological abuse was inflicted in the form of restraint and reward, and I was forced against my will to attend these institutions from a very early age. I'll never forget my first day at 'Infants', age four, screaming and running round the playground with teachers chasing me. Disinterested, dissuaded and very distracted, eventually any hope of being taught about the truth of life was dead. I resigned from the institution and took the path of the seeking into my own hands. I then discovered there was little difference between mainstream education, where the dominant pedagogy is still based on top-down information processing, and management corporations based largely on capitalist ideology, modernity and western individualism.

Freire suggests that holistic education is only possible through the reflective action called praxis, a combination of thought and action, where students and teachers 'reflect simultaneously on themselves and world without dichotomising this reflection from action, and thus establish an authentic form of thought and action' (Freire, 1972, p. 56).

William Isaacs's *Dialogue and the Art of Thinking Together* (1999) is also a landmark testimony of applications of dialogue – at the multinational, corporate level. Yet even now at a quarter of a century old, this return could appear as wishful thinking in the context of competitive and fragmented organisations and social systems. 'School years are the best years of your life' one older boy once repeated to me, as if schools were places of equity, insight, sharing, reflective learning and fun! Listening to the news in the adult world, meanwhile, I became desensitised to the word *dialogue*, as self-elected leaders in the Middle East continued to litter speeches with lies while taking many people deeper into hell with them as they still do.

As an adult I came to realise most people are suspicious of each other and of silence too. In our busy world it's too easy to continue to speak for its own sake, rather than being reflective and silent with one another. Our minds continue in their task of perpetually looking for something or someone to occupy, to calculate and formulate and quantify, using the senses then reflecting this busyness outwardly, avoiding looking at the uncomfortable questions deeper within. We find people talking everywhere – in the street, at school, at work, in shops, on buses, in pubs and restaurants holding drinks while shouting at and above each other. Everywhere people seem to be producing a cacophony of voices exclaiming, opinionating, protesting, debating, conflicting and warring. Silence is used as a weapon too.

Choosing silence in a conversation is a radical stance. A young student in one of my art classes wrote on the personal mandala she'd created, 'I am really not good with words'. My drive is to give others the opportunity and the right to be silent for a while, to allow for a deeper, truer voice to emerge, to bring them back to a state of unity with life, with creation itself. People need the right to be nothing and be reminded of that. People also need each other, not othering, and that's where it gets complicated.

The search for communion and joint learning led me to want to explore the heart of dialogue.

There's a widespread assumption of what dialogue is and what it constitutes. Dialogue isn't two people on a film script, nor is it discussing or debating. Dialogue is made from the Greek words *dia*, meaning 'across' or 'between', and *legein*, meaning 'meaning'.

Renowned quantum scientist-philosopher Professor David Bohm tried to develop an experimental approach to language – a 'new mode' of using existing languages – which he called the rheomode – from the Greek 'rheo-' to flow. This approach was based on his thesis that it might be possible for the syntax and grammatical form of language to be changed by 'allowing the verb rather than the noun to play a primary role' (Bohm, 1980, p. 30). He argued that our language is far too object-oriented or noun-based, and that is making us see a world of static objects instead of dynamic processes.

THE SEEDS OF AUTISM DIALOGUE

The Autism Dialogue Approach was first initiated by me and Professor Liz Milne at the University of Sheffield's Autism Research Lab in 2017. We conceived it as a way to interrogate thinking, generate insight and address what we saw as severe fragmentation in the field of autism. It was also a personal enquiry, so the learning was experiential from the outset. I have to credit Dr Richard Smith at Sheffield Adult Autism and Neurodevelopmental Services for making me feel welcome at their talking support groups and moreover, suggesting I contact Liz about my idea in the first place.

As I began to bring together groups, it was crucial to develop a methodology which included the full, dynamic range of autistic experience in theory, research and practice and practice-based research interventions, to become truly participatory. I wondered if genuine co-design and participatory research could have a profound effect on the way theory development and diagnostic procedures are formulated and tested. Outcome data could be collated and used to help inform dialogue practitioners in collaborative cycles, closing the research to practice gap. It was clear that holistic approaches should support an open culture of autistic knowledge creation and transfer, perhaps even empowering some autistic individuals to adopt autism as a difference to be celebrated, choosing identification over diagnosis. It also felt like edgy work and as an artist, I was never quite sure when the work would be completed.

Dialogue is about meaning-making. Sensory, neural, cognitive and social input, when experienced at incompatible speeds and amounts can result in frightening and immobilising experiences in autistic people. In Autism Dialogue, one of our practices is to slow down the pace of the conversation and reduce the input from the environment. Another is to suspend our assumptions. Canadian artist Erin Manning attempted to address autistic perception as 'the direct perception of the forming of experience' (Manning, 2018, para 4), which correlates with a lack of filtering and relatively 'slow' processing speeds in autism. The early Autism Dialogues indicated there could be an impact on a much wider scale, transferable to other areas where there are issues with sensitivity to experience, meaning-making and fragmentation.

Society is far from whole and rather fragmented. We know this through terms like silo-mentality and the rich-poor divide. So one could ask why there is an ontological tension between those with neurological differences and a polarisation of autistic and non-autistic. In this light, we could forgive those who imagined for too long that the 'autism spectrum' is some sort of linear grading system instead of a multidimensional galaxy of traits and characteristics. We could ask, does the so-called 'predominant neurotype' (Beardon, 2018) even exist and how can that be proved? And if it does, why then does it seek to dominate and support these polarising tendencies at the same time? How and why do our brains even decide there's a duplicity? These are some of the things I've always wondered about. Damian Milton puts it simply: 'a dominant normalising agenda has led to the silencing of the autistic voice in knowledge production and community awareness' (Milton, 2012).

In the field of autism, I haven't found a clearer explanation for this division than in Lori Hogenkamp's 'peripheral minds' framework, and her stress adaptation theory of autism (Hogenkamp, 2018). She basically advocates for when we used to live in more traditional societies, where the 'peripheral minds' (unusual, creative, inventive etc.) would not just be accepted, but seen as essential for a healthy whole community. Hogenkamp identifies as autistic and her work demonstrates a deep enquiry into the nature of *autos*. This theory and similar works are pertinent and in Part 2 of this book I highlight other autistic-led theories which support the need and benefits of a dialogic praxis, from a holistic perspective. Furthermore, the neurodiversity paradigm has enabled us to frame holistically the incredible myriad of human minds, never one ever identical to another. For an opposing view, that of the dangers of human eugenics, one can read Steve Silberman's 'NeuroTribes' (Silberman, 2015) which contains a detailed exploration of the legacy of autism, wherein Hans Asperger's story is revealed as slightly more nuanced than simply as a Nazi collaborator, as many painted him. It's a complicated legacy, and still evolving.

Even most autistic-led autism theories seem to define and support autism as real in the concrete sense. Autism culture attempts to reclaim autism, but one thing I've learned from listening to hundreds of autistic people is that in taking any singular position – whether medically, socially or politically – we risk reinforcing our polarising tendencies, empowering the dominating forces of autism pathology, so the deficit narratives get louder and society digs its heels in further. The human brain seeks to name and categorise, that's its function. Dialogue aims to equalise and dissolve binary dynamics, which is why it works best in a circle. I've been wondering when we will be able to create a circle of little circular Zoom faces on our screens instead of boxes in rows. Meanwhile, you can drag someone you want to hear more from, or identify with, to the top of the screen, if you don't mind removing yourself from the default position!

Words can get in the way of true meaning-making conversation. Dialogue attempts to engage directly with consciousness. Bohm proposed a 'Theory of the Implicate Order' (Bohm, 1980), which, by a cosmic process of unfolding and enfolding, treats the totality of existence as an unbroken whole, and recognises consciousness as always coming into being. Our sacred wisdom traditions and indigenous peoples have always reflected this and Bohm, truly a modern mystic, way ahead of his time, was honoured by the Dalai Lama and Krishnamurti. During an interview for the American Institute of Physics (Wilkins, 1986), Bohm recounts a story of when he was a child, jumping stones across a river and relating it to the flow of thinking – an early description of the quantum leap, which was the start of his enquiry into the flow of thought and experience. Try it. Stop your flow of thinking right now and become aware that everything in this moment has never happened before and never will again. And on we go again.

Western science and the dominating anthropocentric mindset aims to dismantle the miracle of inter-being and eternal unfolding-enfolding of life, but it cannot, for 'science' is another manifestation of that life. 'Science' is already simultaneously the observer, the observed and the observing, leading us finally to consciousness, which has already come into being as soon as 'discovered'. Quantum scientists will forever grapple with existence by drawing long sums on blackboards and searching for the 'God particle' underground in giant circular tunnels. Our perception and understanding of the world are viewed through desperately fragmented wastelands of positive knowledge, advanced by our esteemed universities and upon which society's policies so precariously balance. I don't mean to be cynical, just redressing the balance a bit, because something's rotten in the state of things.

In autism, there exists multiple conflicting ideologies and viewpoints (at the systemic level) and false dichotomies, yet there are no biomarkers in autism. It is a social construct and its meaning is medically dominated. Dominant autism practices are rife with ableism and normalcy narratives; polarising tendencies result in social movements becoming self-alienating too. In health research, the time-lag between research evidence and subsequent translation into practice is estimated to be 17 years (Morris et al., 2011; Robinson, 2020). Evidence-based practice is difficult because 'quality of life' and definitions of 'success/values' are too often situated within a dominant fix-it culture which defines success as 'normalisation'.

Quality of life, a complex concept with varied definitions, is constructed according to the Australian Centre on Quality of Life's framework (2017, para. 1):

> *Quality of life is both objective and subjective.* These two dimensions encompass several domains, which collectively define the construct. Objective domains are assessed through culturally relevant measures of wellbeing, while subjective domains are evaluated through satisfaction-based questions.

A recent study on the Personal Wellness Index (PWI) was commissioned by London South Bank University and has emerged as an effective tool for assessing quality of life and wellbeing, gaining positive reception from both neurotypical and neurodivergent participants. This research is pioneering due to its creation of a concise, multidimensional measure of wellbeing applicable across the UK population. The tool now allows for meaningful comparisons between different groups and the societal average using more nuanced criteria. It is a significant contribution to the international quality of life database (R. Mills, personal communication, 20 May 2024).

FIRST EXPERIMENTS WITH DIALOGUE

I took part in the first Bohm Dialogue sessions held at Sheffield Hallam University, during my final year of a Contemporary Fine Art degree, invited by Hester Reeve and Helen Blejerman. We were to see these as a kind of 'crit' (critique of art) session but without the art. Thinking and language became the tools of expression to be brought forth into the space as our 'canvas'. Open and inquisitive students and locals from the art scene gravitated to our basement room to join the experiment; most were mature students but occasionally younger, more reflective and quieter ones came. We sat for a few hours, generating insight together. With a light introduction from our tutor, it was at times awkward and a bit uncomfortable and yet always revealing for each other, as we discovered when we 'checked out' at the end. During one session I had the experience of witnessing a large bubble of intuitive energy hovering over our circle, enveloping us all at the same time, accompanied by a feeling of total congruence, which Helen felt too, describing it as love. I knew then that I would always somehow be involved with Dialogue.

Immediately after graduating, with the assistance of an open-minded project manager who later became my wife, I transformed a local gallery into a learning centre and became their first education manager. I hired my own studio next door, to design creativity programmes for the gallery. The first programmes were all about self-discovery and identity for local refugees and home-schooled children, and I brought in other artist-educators for a broader range of input, to share their knowledge and co-facilitate workshops. We began to experiment using dialogue along with storytelling to enhance a sense of self and for the adults, their employability. We called one programme 'Creating Identities'. Some years later I discovered I had been applying techniques found more commonly in the fields of auto-ethnography and narrative coaching. Although our small team was funded by the European Regional Development Fund, because the work was experimental, at times my self-esteem suffered, even at times feeling a hint of 'playing God' as I moved into my new role, grappling with an enormous sense of potential and the enjoyment of structured conversation and process control. I learned experientially the importance of the 'contract' and the understanding/agreement between facilitators, organisers, and delegates. This applied self-awareness turned out to be my early fine tuning as facilitator.

Contracted by Leeds Artforms to design and run 'My Sacred Identity' sessions in several schools, I felt privileged to work with young minds who responded well, especially to the sections of generative dialogue, storytelling and mindfulness meditation. As an artist-educator, I was aiming to unite self-discovery, peer-learning, communication and creative expression with dialogic encounters, to make a case for how such environments can be useful for the common good, and those young minds were to me always surprisingly receptive and an honour to witness. Affirmed to me mostly by the children I worked with, who it appeared were as yet relatively unchallenged by modernity, I realised that in dialogue one could understand, in a small but important way, how vital it is to see the universe as an undivided whole; to see it, embody it, experience it and really know it.

My search for unification and harmony since childhood has taken me through many spiritual doors, one known as non-duality, a term borrowed from Eastern mysticism and translated from the Sanskrit word 'Advaita'. Perhaps more easily understood as 'unity of existence' or interconnectedness, it is present in most, if not all of the world's great wisdom traditions, found in Zen, Taoism, Sufism, Buddhism, Hinduism etc. and is a familiar concept in ecology, biodiversity, neurodiversity and so on. Crucially for the topic of this book, the concept of intersubjectivity, when more than one subject relates to another, is an extension of the idea of an undivided whole. From the social perspective, this supports our need for relationships and shared human experiences, which fosters societal harmony. Therefore non-duality, along with other spiritual terms, may be perceived not as something esoteric and out of reach, but as a refreshing reminder of our true origin. A broad field of vision, incorporating all wisdom traditions – east and west – is necessary if we are going to embrace a truly holistic, enquiring approach to the scientific practice of dialogue and an inclusive ontological perspective of autism.

In this book you will be guided from the philosophical underpinnings of autism and dialogue to practical suggestions for experimenting with techniques in various settings – whether in groups or pairs, or in community or organisational contexts. You might be inspired to start an 'Autism Dialogue' group in your own community, becoming a catalyst for others to do the same. I ask you to remember that what we did, how we did it and what we discovered, will differ from how you might choose to approach and experience this framework. As long as you are kind and follow the general idea, the Autism Dialogue Approach is yours to experiment with. No one can own it, as much as anyone can own the concepts of autism or dialogue.

A HANDBOOK

Despite being titled a handbook, this is not a step-by-step guide to a new methodology. Rather, it is an invitation to journey with me through about eight years of 'Autism Dialogues', culminating in case studies, insights, and suggestions. It includes autobiographical elements that reflect my experiences and serve as examples for applying the approach. My aim is to inspire creativity in you, particularly if you work in fields such as creative social practice, education, cognitive sciences, healthcare, or therapy. This book is also for scholars and students of disability studies, social studies, or anyone interested in engaging with autism more thoughtfully and compassionately.

The Autism Dialogue Approach takes a holistic view, encompassing the humanistic, social, systemic, and spiritual dimensions of autism, selfhood and our existence. It provides support through talking about creative ideas, personal experience and even problems. It provides insights for autistic people and anyone working relationally with adults, many of whom may be autistic. You see, as autism is invisible (and there's no autism biology to be found either) you never know who is autistic. You might think you know, but that's different.

This book welcomes you into the ongoing dialogue around autism, a dynamic and mysterious human phenomenon that is always in flux. The conversation around autism in the broader social context is ongoing, and this book is but a small contribution to that evolving dialogue. In 2017 I attended the inaugural meeting of the Academy of Professional Dialogue (AoPD). There I was informed by Peter Garrett, a co-author (along with David Bohm and Donald Factor) of the seminal paper 'Dialogue – A Proposal' (Bohm et al., 1991), that no one had yet applied Dialogue in a therapeutic setting. While the Autism Dialogue Approach is not necessarily therapeutic, this revelation suggested that it could indeed be considered innovative. However, as my work did not include a systematic search for related literature, I remain open to feedback and welcome contributions from others exploring similar approaches.

As I wrote these words, I discovered a friend and mentor, author of NeuroTribes, Steve Silberman had passed away, which caused me great sadness not only because he was a fabulously colourful and likeable man, but because of what he stood for as an ally to the autistic community. During an interview I conducted with Steve he said: 'Reading your paper on autism dialogues, it seemed like exactly the sort of steps that need to be taken' (Dialogica, 2019).

As we walk precariously and yet hopefully robustly into the future of autism, it's increasingly apparent the world really does need Dialogue. Author and researcher Nick Chown said to me, 'There is a long way to go before we are seen as a minority like ethnic, religious, and sexual minorities. Your Dialogue events will get us there a little more quickly' (personal communication, 4 September 2019).

We must rediscover the timeless principles for creative collaboration that transcend capital and hierarchical structures, embracing a politics of the soul, which values every individual's unique contribution to the whole. This book is an invitation to engage in that dialogue, to listen deeply, and to participate in the co-creation of a more compassionate and inclusive world.

I use a capital D in Dialogue, to pay respect to this amazing word and to delineate it from its other meanings, of which there are many.

HOW TO READ THIS BOOK

The book is in three parts. Part I frames my personal, academic and professional history. You will begin to learn, and in some cases unlearn, about what dialogue is and what autism is, in order to get into the spirit of enquiry – bringing you into the dialogue, as it were.

In Part II, after the essential Chapter 5, you could go straight to Chapters 9–11 for my practice experiences and some guidance at the heart of the approach and this handbook. Chapter 10 assumes you want to learn how to run Dialogues, and is a 'must read' from a professional, safe practice point of view. Chapter 6 explains the key concepts and terminology of autism as a way of being and covers sensory sensitivity, masking and communication in contexts of society, to equip you with some basics in preparation for Dialogues in Autism. My perspective on neurodiversity is quite radical so please read it at some point, and when you're ready, go back to Chapter 7, the most research-heavy chapter of the book, which dives deeper into social science and philosophical concerns and optimism.

Part III, 'Wider Contexts', broadens the enquiry and I try to simplify some of the wider concepts to help unite them, such as therapy, spirituality and culture. Did you know 'intersection' is the American word for the English 'crossroads', and intersectionality is simply a metaphor for someone who 'stands' at the centre and is multiply disadvantaged by oncoming discrimination (traffic)? It's sometimes a matter of just standing back from the noise in order to find out what people and big words and concepts really mean. Dialogue is very practical and this means dissecting words and meanings, and using etymology, so together we can find out their possible uses. I've heard many people realise that good therapy and coaching is simply about connecting and so if you work in this area, please study this chapter. Dialogue provides space, which is good for autistic people and one of my favourite topics; I explore this further in the chapter on spirituality. Mindful awareness and spirituality are other terms taken to be something complicated, but are really just about default human nature. I tie up the practice of Dialogue with the benefits and practicalities of space-clearing and meditation for autistic wellbeing and collective meaning-making. There are case examples included as appendices for you to be further inspired!

REFERENCES

Australian Centre on Quality of Life. (2017). What is quality of life? Retrieved from www.acqol.com.au/about

Beardon, L. (2018). Is autism a disorder? Retrieved from https://blogs.shu.ac.uk/autism/2018/07/17/is-autism-a-disorder/#

Bohm, D. (1980). *Wholeness and the Implicate Order*. Routledge and Kegan Paul.

Bohm, D., Factor, D. & Garrett, P. (1991). *Dialogue – a proposal*. Academy of Professional Dialogue. Retrieved from https://aofpd.org/library/public-resources/dialogue-a-proposal/

Dialogica. (2019). Steve Silberman interview, bestselling author of *Neurotribes, The Legacy of Autism* [Video file]. Retrieved from https://youtu.be/EvrR5-3_zAY

Freire, P. (1972). *Pedagogy of the Oppressed*. Penguin Books.

Hogenkamp, L. (2018). Is autism a stress adaptation of neurodivergent neurotypes? Retrieved from https://peripheralmindsofautism.com/2018/04/17/is-autism-a-stress-adaptation/

Isaacs, W. (1999). *Dialogue and the Art of Thinking Together: A Pioneering Approach to Communicating in Business and in Life*. Currency.

Manning, E. (2018). Histories of violence: neurodiversity and the policing of the norm. Retrieved from https://lareviewofbooks.org/article/histories-of-violence-neurodiversity-and-the-policing-of-the-norm

Milton, D. (2012). The normalisation agenda and the psycho-emotional disablement of autistic people. Presented at CeDR Disability Studies Conference, Lancaster, UK, 11–13 September.

Morris, Z. S., Wooding, S. & Grant, J. (2011). The answer is 17 years, what is the question: understanding time lags in translational research. *Journal of the Royal Society of Medicine*, 104(12), 510–520.

Robinson, T., et al. (2020). Bridging the research–practice gap in healthcare: a rapid review of research translation centres in England and Australia. *Health Res Policy Sys*, 18(117). https://doi.org/10.1186/s12961-020-00621-w

Silberman, S. (2015). *Neurotribes: The Legacy of Autism and How to Think Smarter about People Who Think Differently*. Allen & Unwin.

Wilkins, M. (1986). David Bohm – Session I [interview with David Bohm by Maurice Wilkins]. Retrieved from www.aip.org/history-programs/niels-bohr-library/oral-histories/32977-1

CHAPTER 2

Autism as a way of being

....

Autism is a way of being. It is pervasive; it colours every experience, every sensation, perception, thought, emotion, and encounter, every aspect of existence. It is not possible to separate the autism from the person – and if it were possible, the person you'd have left would not be the same person you started with.

(Sinclair, 1993, para. 5)

Autism is an evolving construct. My writing this and you reading it is all part of the continual unfolding process of defining it. We are literally making it up as we go along. Feel free to go and look up current definitions of autism, autism spectrum disorder, autism spectrum condition, the autisms (plural) etc. I make no apologies for the amount of introspection below and elsewhere in this book. I've opened my personal exploration somewhat, for you and the world to read in this book, because that's what I do best, so please accept the autobiographical nature of various sections. Of course, I've worked heavily on the wider context, with support, without which it wouldn't have got past several peer-review stages and finally into print!

DISCOVERY JOURNEY

After I graduated from university, the government arts cuts came in. It was 2011. Over the following five years I launched several small businesses, experiencing temporary success followed by their respective failures, one at a catastrophic level. Having had enough of living at that pace and confusion, always returning to existential crisis in trying to work out the system and my place in it and getting increasingly confused, I went to the doctor. As a default square peg in a round hole, I urgently needed answers.

I already knew I was sensitive when I picked up a battered copy of Elaine Aron's *Highly Sensitive Person* (Aron, 2017) in a charity shop. 'Highly sensitive person'

(HSP) is now a medicalised term. My father had already said he thought I might have Asperger's, as a nurse once told him she thought he had it, and as it's genetic, he let me know. Some years later it was clear to me it was the source of most of his problems. I did the online autism test, and I came out with a high score, so I wrote out a list of the things that bothered me, such as low tolerance of people and sensory sensitivities as well as a number of weird quirky things that I can live with or that I actually like about myself. Handing it to my GP, I asked him what he thought, upon which he referred me to the NHS adult autism service.

A few months later I sat in a dimly lit, grey-walled room, staring blankly back at the psychologist. After three sessions totalling nearly six hours of questioning, I was back for the final outcome. She announced, 'You meet the criteria for Asperger Syndrome' and left a pause. A rush of thoughts rose in my head, along with a sense of amusement and disbelief. 'Wrong person. What the hell do they know about me?' She continued, 'Some people react at this point, perhaps with a feeling of relief or upset.' Watching me closely, she added, 'And sometimes people might have a few tears.' Suddenly emotions coursed through my body and tears broke in a strange mixture of relief that I'd won a prize, and the realisation in being told I was basically a bit of a dud. I put my face in my hands and deep down the question stirred, 'Why is life so damn unpredictable?' A seed of ableism had been planted and was taking root.

A long explanatory letter was handed to me. It recounted a lot of the stuff about childhood trauma I'd experienced, which was shocking to read back to myself. I had some denial mixed in but I quickly took my new medical diagnosis with a pinch of salt and a dose of healthy scepticism. Over the following months, I struggled and grappled with the complexities, many of them historic, existential, systemic, social and of course, spiritual and cosmological. A few months later, a letter dropped on the doormat with the bonus news that I met the criteria for ADHD.

On a mission to get a deeper understanding of 'this autistic thing', I enrolled on a master's degree in Autism Spectrum at Sheffield Hallam University. I lasted just a year because I started to learn some uncomfortable truths about medical research, eugenics and electric shock vest control and besides, I wanted to launch the dialogues in the community and get on with the job of directly helping people. I reflected deeply and wrote on the fragmentation within the definitions of autism, with its variety of opinion camps and conflicting ideologies. I learned about neurodiversity, savants and superpowers; deficit models and predominant neurotype narratives, forced behavioural therapy, global clinical research and conformist programmes delivered by autism charities, mostly in the US. I was particularly interested in these complex relational issues, all the while having a sense of how much kindness and harmony is missing in the world.

Most urgent for me was the unravelling and consolidating of almost fifty years under this new lens. I did a lot of unravelling. I came to realise that I had often placed more importance on specific things than most other people, sometimes beyond what was necessary, ranging from observances of the tiniest things in my vision and thoughts to major world events and planetary phenomena, and most particularly with relationships and humans. Social interactions, personal relationships, brief exchanges both verbal and physical and even the anticipation of potential meetings could trigger anxiety, worry, excitement, puzzlement and sometimes deep existential enquiry. This enquiry was most pronounced in the relationship with myself, my environment and my meaning to existence within it. For most people, this can basically be summed up in the common question 'What's my place in society?' and most people just seemed to get on with it. Special interests (increasingly nowadays referred to as focussed interests) is a common trait among autistics. Mine was and still is the question of 'What is the self and why do I exist?' I was sure people used to ask that more in the '80s but I had no choice but to continue asking: 'Why are we here?' I still can't think of a better question worth asking. Okay, maybe 'Who am I?' – also known as the practice of Atma Vichara – which therapist Nic Higham describes like this: 'There is no doubt if you sincerely pursued the question "Who am I?" rigorously, you would come to the conclusion that you cannot be defined as the body, the mind, the thoughts or the events that you experience' (Higham, 2022).

I realised there were also benefits to my brain placing more importance on things than necessary. An overstimulated mental position can be detrimental but also very productive. Socially, I was aware that some people, sometimes might instil in me acute anxiety, whereas the same person in another situation could actually make me feel comfortable and even empowered. This I've come to know as hyper-empathy. In the early stages of my autism discovery, relationships were all quite unpredictable. Had they always been this way? I wondered. Experimenting and being more aware while looking through this new lens, I realised experientially that a social exchange is a two-way relationship and not something we should ever take for granted. However, there was a certain something in me that was markedly different to the standard, typical person. I was only dimly aware that western scientific medicine had categorised the condition called autism quite apart from other mental conditions. The DSM (Diagnostic Statistical Manual) is littered with deficit language and enough to really bring everyone down.

Autism is an innate part of a person, so it is not subject to 'cure'. It is impossible to separate the individual and their autistic experience from society and yet, in returning to the origins of the modern autism construct, Hans Asperger stated: 'The autist is only himself … and is not an active member of a greater organism which he is influenced by and which he influences constantly' (Asperger, 1991). Yet autism cannot be found, like the self, there is no biomarker.

'Who is creating the science?' was my new burning question. Dr Luke Beardon from Sheffield Hallam University has placed autistic outcomes as totally intrinsic to the environment (Beardon, 2018), which seemed to me contrary to Asperger's primitive view of an 'isolated self'. Meanwhile, the neurodiversity movement is a testament to the power of collective consciousness:

> There needs to be greater recognition that the autism identity is a social construction with the potential to constrain and degrade. In identity terminology, individuals need to be enabled to identify with a group that is perceived as constructive and empowering rather than detrimental and limiting.
>
> *(MacLeod, Lewis & Robertson, 2013, p. 47)*

I had always grappled, not just with identity or community belonging, but with the polarising of the individual and the collective. At those original autism assessments, I'd asked the neuropathologist about Advaita Vedanta and non-dual consciousness. Of course, she knew nothing about it – and duly made a note about my asking the question on her clipboard. I was now intrigued and excited by the potential for a huge new enquiry. All these different emerging cognitive sciences, systemic polarising tendencies and conflicting ideologies, just within the west was mind-boggling and intriguing. And looking east there was nothing; indeed, some cultures don't even have a word for anxiety let alone autism.

I was soon glad to have been ticketed with this mysterious, subtle and yet profound condition, because not only could I now begin to manage my personality and mentality from a more informed, empowered position, at least within the current societal context, but I had something to think about and perhaps even make a career out of.

In dialogue micro-communities, autistic people could be empowered by positively identifying with their own community but also becoming more familiar with those in their other community – including everyone in the new neurodiverse universe.

This might relieve pressure from private and public healthcare services. Autism Dialogue could be used in organisational development, at the interface between researchers, healthcare staff, service users and their support networks, and as a front-line offering via community doctors in 'social-prescribing'. I decided to trust this new lifeworld perspective and contribute to its evolution, feeling that the correct management would bring more quality to my life and relating to the world.

Going internally deeper into notions of authenticity, before I knew anything about the concept of autistic 'masking', I wrote a few thoughts in my diary, about what I called 'the glass mask':

> We all wear our personality traits (masks) and behave in special ways for different people, in different circumstances and in different social contexts and cultures. A measure of this would be to ask yourself how relaxed and open you were with the neighbour you don't really get along with or a store assistant. We have social norms and the way you behave with your spouse won't be the same way you behave with your work colleagues. These masks, which are a major part of our psychology, we design not to disguise our total self but to 'play a part' of ourselves in order to make things run more smoothly and efficiently, to get what we want and at the same time help maintain a functioning society. The glass mask is a term that I came up with to describe the sensation or phenomenon of the continuous mask wearing that someone like me might use to cope and maintain smooth functioning with the whole world at large. With the very unpredictable and usually heightened sensory stimulation an 'autistic person' experiences, a constant coping mechanism develops; a glass mask. This could imply that the person, in wearing a mask constantly, is never their real self (whatever that may be) but I argue that is not the case. You can 'see the person' through the mask (and they can see you of course) but

as the passive observer, you may notice a slight unusualness about them; an odd, perhaps ungrounded-ness or intensity as the mask (and the person) does its best to maintain equilibrium in the sensory (and social) circus, which is the mind of the autistic and by extension, multidirectional social interactions. For the person wearing the glass mask, a struggle may be taking place. The unpredictable fluctuations of the levels of sensory input being received and transmitted by the brain mean constant guardedness is needed. Removing the mask would leave the person open to reveal extraordinary levels of brain activity, which could damage the circumstance and upset the relationship. Leaving it on, strange and usually very tiring as it may be, they know they aren't being fully themselves. This is the dichotomy of the mask; it is a simple yet profound coping mechanism, which is constant, but for some of the time (when brain activity is stable) it can be an encumbrance. Behind the transparency, looking out, there is a real person and like many people, often cautious and vulnerable. Mask-wearers are usually very perceptive and have the ability to spot other mask-wearers; they hold sincerity and truth in very high, even holy regard.

The beauty of the mask is also its transparency. I've realised if you look at an autistic person closely in a certain way at the right moment, you might see through the mask and be rewarded in seeing a real, sincere and special (as we all are in reality) human being. In so doing you may even play a part in aiding them, for just a moment, to discard the glass mask.

I had self-insight. Over many years I'd done a lot of work in the form of spiritual effort, formal training and self-discovery workshops. So far, I'd trained in support work, chaplaincy, mindfulness, victim-offender mediation, vipassana, personal development, coaching and counselling. And now, as an 'expert by experience', I was nurturing a strong sense of how education and self (*autos*) discovery could be much more cohesive.

It was during the university Autism course that I discovered the complex journey from autism theory and practice to the autistic experience is extremely complex and long. I reached a new understanding and a certain amount of gratitude for being able to contribute in a small way to the evolution of autism practice – by this apparent being of autistic. I had also accepted that I struggled to act fully within the paradigm of our society, as in doing so, I sacrificed psychological wellbeing and experienced anxiety and heightened emotion. My final essay was the very real dilemma of an autistic person studying autism within a predominantly non-autistic system and a clear example of the main presiding challenge. I opened myself to further disabling society as I entertained excessive thinking within the current societal paradigm. Was I perpetuating the myth by taking part in it? At the same time I thought by remaining true to myself, I could not be socially disabled, as I was not a member of that disabling (aspect of) society. I thought about the limits of the social model of disability and Autism is as much of a construct as social disability, which simply assumes our society contributes to disability. A cultural shift is taking place and there's growing evidence that autistic people understand each other in specific ways. Autistic researchers and practitioners are increasing in number and I felt hopeful this will lead to more experience-based research and less mimicking of 'neurotypical' behaviour on both individual and collective levels.

See Appendix 1 for more on Research and Evaluation.

AUTISTIC CULTURE

When meeting an autistic person, we must regard their communication in the context of autistic culture. As we would adapt to a person from any other different cultural background or ethnicity, we should seek to learn about their customs and practices and respectfully adapt our behaviour to suit them.

There is pressure on autistic people in unnamed 'social skills' programmes and approaches, even to use the spoken word, reinforcing messages about normalisation and potentially increasing trauma. Autistic communication and social styles are genuinely different and equally effective, so we can't see autistic people having a communication deficit that needs to be overcome by teaching them social skills or judging them.

Autistic culture respects:

- Little to no eye contact, sometimes
- Transparency and honesty
- Quieter, low-arousal environments and socialising
- Shorthand, streamlined, practical, literal communication
- A preference for thinking in patterns
- Absolute accuracy as a cultural expectation, not being pedantic
- Honesty and fairness
- Not always using spoken words

Autism is also a collective mystery. It is meta-loneliness, a hyper-sensitivity to the pervasiveness of society's socialising and socialism, a fundamental state of anxiety and sensory sensitivity norms and a fundamental inability to conformity, and like PTSD and stress-adaptation, these things adversely affect the nervous system. Surges might create so-called special interests and specific high-level skills. 'We are all a little bit autistic' is unhelpful for those needing support and the specific identity, but perhaps in another way it is true, because we are all connected – we are not just separate individuals. We are linguistic bodies (Di Paolo et al., 2018) that enact and interact with endless factors and essences. We all affect each other as individuals and as one. Autistic people included, affect all other people and environments in turn. Autism is the environment; society is therefore autistic.

Autism as a construct spreads even neurologically through culture and society; it is an ideology in perpetual, cyclic process. Using our skill of viewing objectively is more helpful and purposeful than individual subjects and Bohm's (1980) theories of wholeness have contributed to my personal development and the development of Autism Dialogue, consequently helping participants to become whole and interconnected – communicating with each other, intersubjectively, with that divine, equanimous, interpersonal unity of human being-ness and infinite empathy. Autistic traits along an individual's timeline, pre and post diagnosis, are a study in themselves and as one may contemplate the problem of being told they are autistic by non-autistic science, behaviour-masking and behaviour-influencing cycles of self swirl round the apparent autistic head.

There is apparently an epidemic in autism diagnosis. Referencing the idea of normal, this seems more like a collective neurotic reaction. So it is in the collective, in which we must explore. The autistic mind pushes back, opens into a 'dialogue for one'; an enquiry of self-awareness, creative imagination, language, etymology, embodied cognition, enactivism, activism, social and sacred justice, gestalt perception, symbolism, science, spirituality, anthropology, birth, death, the beyond, congruence, relationship-centred care, participatory sense-making, participatory research, quantum science, neuroepigenetics, ethnography, intersubjectivity, therapy, coaching, non-dual healing, resonance, energy and proximity laws, remote healing, Atma and Brahma, Advaita Vedanta, Atma Vichara, Shaman, Sufi, Tao, Zen, Buddha … God, and baby rabbits.

An autistic person may be well aware of that human journey back to selfhood, to a unified consciousness, yet somehow feel locked into the world of gross form and competing social constructs, reinforced by a sense of self, inadvertently or not. What a nightmare existence, which must surely raise our compassion. It's time for Dialogue!

REFERENCES

Aron, E. N. (2014). *The Highly Sensitive Person: How to Survive and Thrive When the World Overwhelms You*. Thorsons.

Asperger, H. (1991). 'Autistic psychopathy' in childhood. In U. Frith (ed., trans.), *Autism and Asperger syndrome* (pp. 37–92). Cambridge University Press. https://doi.org/10.1017/CBO9780511526770.002 (This chapter is an annotated translation of a German article by Hans Asperger that was published in 1944 in *Archiv für Psychiatrie und Nervenkrankheiten*, 117, 76–136.)

Beardon, L. (2018). Three golden rules for supporting autistic pupils. *TES Magazine*, 7 November. Retrieved from www.tes.com/magazine/archive/three-golden-rules-supporting-autistic-pupils

Bohm, D. (1980). *Wholeness and the Implicate Order*. Routledge & Kegan Paul.

Di Paolo, E., De Jaegher, H. & Cuffari, E. (2018) *Linguistic Bodies: The Continuity between Life and Language*. MIT Press.

Higham, N. (2022). The practice of Atma Vichara by Sri Ramana Maharshi: the wholeness of experience. Retrieved from https://nisargayoga.org/the-practice-of-atma-vichara-by-sri-ramana-maharshi – June 2024

MacLeod, A., Lewis, A. & Robertson, C. (2013), 'Why should I be like bloody Rain Man?!' Navigating the autistic identity. *British Journal of Special Education*, 40, 41–49. https://doi.org/10.1111/1467-8578.12015

Sinclair, J. (1993). Don't mourn for us. Retrieved from www.autreat.com/dont_mourn.html

CHAPTER 3

Dialogue in historical context

Good dialogue helps people find common understanding and purpose, leading to decisions that make sense to everyone involved. It involves expressing views, listening, supporting, and challenging, fostering an appreciation for diversity and enabling sustainable, participatory change.

Dialogue aims to transform not only how we think but also how we reflect on our thinking. Bohm, who was greatly troubled from a young age, perceived fragmentation in thinking suggesting, 'In a dialogue, there is no attempt to gain points, or to make your particular view prevail. Rather, whenever any mistake is discovered on the part of anybody, everybody gains' (Bohm, 1996). We've been taught to divide and categorise the world, yet we then behave as if these divisions don't exist, assuming that our thoughts are an accurate reflection of reality. Bohm's ideas were heavily influenced by quantum theory, which suggests that the observer and the observed are not truly separate and Bohm's own magnum opus in the field was *Wholeness and the Implicate Order* (Bohm, 1980). What we perceive is shaped by our own observation. Through collective dialogue, where a large group speaks together in a circle, this shift in perception occurs collaboratively.

Isaacs put the problem of thinking thus: 'What you perceive, in other words, is not determined by independent external properties of "parts" of reality, but is a function of the ways in which you try to perceive that reality' (Isaacs, 1996).

I discuss various configurations of Dialogue practice later on. It is a very broad topic and a full appraisal is beyond the scope of this book. I will briefly introduce historical, philosophical, and anthropological perspectives to illuminate the significance of group dialogue and communication, shedding light on traditional societies and their unique approaches to conflict resolution, knowledge transmission, and cultural preservation. More broadly in the context of today's world, I focus on dialogue as the practice of people meeting in person or online, to address collective challenges and growth pertinent to autism and neurodiversity.

Examine the definition of *dialogue* from the Online Etymology Dictionary (n.d.):

> 'Dialogue – c. 1200, 'literary work consisting of a conversation between two or more persons,' from Old French *dialoge* and directly from Latin *dialogus*, from Greek *dialogos* 'conversation, dialogue,' related to *dialogesthai* 'converse,' from *dia* 'across, between' (see *dia-*) + *legein* 'to speak' (from PIE root **leg-* (1) 'to collect, gather,' with derivatives meaning 'to speak (to "pick out words")')'.
>
> The sense was extended by c. 1400 to 'a conversation between two or more persons.' The mistaken belief that it can mean only 'conversation between two persons' is from confusion of *dia-* and *di-* (1); as early as 1532, *trialogue* appears needlessly for 'a conversation between three persons.' Also compare *quadrilogue* 'dialogue of four speakers' (late 15c.), in the title of the English translation of '*Quadrilogue invectif*,' which consists of an allegorical dialogue between the Three Estates and a personified France.
>
> A word that has been used for 'conversation between two persons' and cannot mean otherwise is the hybrid *duologue* (1864).

TRADITIONAL COMMUNITIES AND SOCIETIES

As Bohm intimated below, anthropologists and sociologists suggest that the ideal size for a human community is around 100 to 150 people, a concept known as 'Dunbar's Number' from British anthropologist Robin Dunbar, who found that human brain capacity allows us to maintain stable social relationships with about this many individuals (Dunbar & Shultz, 2007).

> Some time ago there was an anthropologist who lived for a long while with a North American tribe. It was a small group of about fifty people ... Now, from time to time that tribe met like this in a circle. They just talked and talked and talked, apparently to no purpose. They made no decisions. There was no leader. And everybody could participate. There may have been wise men or wise women who were listened to a bit more – the older ones – but everybody could talk. The meeting went on, until it finally seemed to stop for no reason at all and the group dispersed. Yet after that, everybody seemed to know what to do, because they understood each other so well. Then they could get together in smaller groups and do something or decide things.
>
> *(Bohm, 1996)*

In such communities, everyone knows one another, which fosters trust, cooperation, and accountability – key factors in maintaining a healthy and cohesive society. Communities of this size also create a balance between social connection and privacy. They are large enough to provide diverse skills, support systems, and resources, yet small enough to prevent feelings of isolation or excessive competition. In these groups, individuals can participate in meaningful dialogue, ensuring that everyone's needs are heard and considered, which reduces social stress and promotes a sense of belonging. This scale of community living is thought to reflect how humans evolved in tribal societies, where the close-knit nature of relationships allowed for greater social harmony and collective resilience.

Additionally, smaller communities with this structure are more adept at managing conflict and fostering cooperation, as individuals can regularly interact face-to-face. This size is optimal for maintaining complex social bonds, ensuring that each person has a role and a place in the group.

Autistic social scientist Lori Hogenkamp (2018) proposes that traditional societies, which were organised into smaller, more inclusive communities, allowed for a natural integration of diverse cognitive and behavioural profiles. These smaller, cooperative groups fostered adaptive mechanisms that embraced individuals with 'peripheral minds' – those who may have had neurodivergent traits but played essential roles in the group's survival and innovation.

Individuals on the cognitive periphery had heightened skills in creativity, problem-solving, and resilience, which benefited the whole community. Dialogue played a crucial role in maintaining social cohesion. It allowed for the expression of different viewpoints and the mutual regulation of stress, as community members supported and challenged one another. This communication helped ensure that all members, regardless of their neurocognitive profiles, were valued, thus contributing to a healthy and inclusive society.

The framework of neurodiversity today still draws upon these ancient principles, where the unique adaptive responses of neurodivergent individuals are seen as valuable contributions to societal resilience and long-term sustainability. Hogenkamp's Evolutionary-Stress Framework (Center for Adaptive Stress, 2022) further suggests that neurodiversity is an inherent part of human evolution, with peripheral minds serving vital functions within the broader adaptive network of human communities.

DIALOGUE AND INDIGENOUS SOCIETIES

Typical conversational modes such as discussion and debate are often competitive and as a result views of autism can be polarised, providing little scope for nuanced discussion and active listening. Dialogue has the potential to make a positive difference in the way autism is understood by all. A principle of Dialogue is that individuals try to build upon others' ideas so that new knowledge and a collective understanding can be formed. In this respect, Dialogue plays an important role in accelerating discussion via a common understanding and increasing social and professional cohesion of the whole autism arena and beyond.

Humanity has a rich tapestry of dialogue, and by extension, the oral traditions have always been a primary mode of communication. But it doesn't really have that much to do with speaking! The word dialogue, in essence, can be translated from the Greek as 'through-meaning' emphasising the cultivation of a deep sense of interconnectedness and harmony, preserving cultural heritage through historical narratives and traditional wisdom. Indigenous societies and religious and spiritual communities, which have thrived for centuries across the globe, have developed intricate systems of group dialogue and communication that are central to their personal growth and cultural, social, and ecological resilience. Through storytelling, songs, and rituals, we pass down knowledge from one generation to the next. The oral traditions are the lifeblood, not only binding communities but also ensuring the continuity of their cultural identity.

Native American tribes are renowned for their sophisticated system of governance, rooted in group dialogue and consensus-building. The Great Law of Peace of the Iroquois Confederacy (also known as the Haudenosauneeir) dates back over 1,000 years, and helped establish their principles of collective decision-making and mediation. In South Africa, the San people have community gatherings where everyone has a voice and decisions are made collectively, ensuring the equitable distribution of resources, fostering social cohesion and sustaining harmonious existence in a challenging environment. The Maori people of New Zealand embody the worldview of 'whanaungatanga', emphasising interconnectedness and unity. The Kogi in Colombia are known for their deep spiritual connection to nature and their dedication to preserving the ecological balance of their territory and through group dialogues and ceremonies, maintaining a complex system of agricultural and ecological knowledge. The Mbuti Pygmies, residing in the rainforests of central Africa, rely on group dialogue and cooperation for their nomadic hunter-gatherer lifestyle.

The Kurds, who are spread across several countries in the Middle East, have a strong tradition of community dialogue and decision-making through assemblies known as *jameels* (women's assemblies). The Druze community has a unique system of community governance that includes councils known as *majalis*. The Hmong of China, Vietnam, Laos and Thailand, The Karen of Myanmar and Thailand, The Yezidis of northern Iraq, The Ryukyuan of the Japanese islands; all of these indigenous communities have traditional forms of dialogue where elders and community members gather to discuss issues and make decisions, usually conducting dialogue in a circle, the representation of unity. Participants are aware that it is only if they are united and whole, facing each other in honesty, that they can truly address their concerns. We will later further explore the significance of the circle gathering in the context of Autism Dialogue.

Traditional and indigenous societies have often managed to preserve their cultures through group dialogue, despite external pressures. Furthermore, the barriers between indigenous and non-indigenous communities are well documented and a source of sorrow and shame for many who seek to promote intercultural dialogues to foster mutual understanding and cooperation.

By continuously discussing their customs, beliefs, and practices, communities adapt to changing circumstances while staying rooted in their cultural heritage. Successful governance relies on robust decision-making processes and group dialogues serve as the cornerstone of governance, ensuring that decisions are made collectively and that the community's voice is heard, providing cultural resilience and firm governance, an approach which fosters a strong sense of ownership and accountability within the community.

For all of these indigenous groups, dialogue plays a pivotal role in their society, in systems of communal decision-making through consensus. Gatherings are instrumental in maintaining social cohesion and preserving their unique cultural practices. Tribal councils serve as platforms where community members can voice their concerns, discuss disputes, and seek consensus-based solutions, dialogues which are often facilitated by respected elders who possess a deep understanding of tribal customs and values, ensuring a fair and just resolution process as well as ensuring the transmission of wisdom from one generation to the next. Sharing ecological wisdom is important to maintain an intimate relationship with the natural surroundings, survival often depending on sustainable resource management and ecological knowledge.

Communalism and a collective sense of self are traditionally valued more than anthropocentrism; a communal worldview places great importance on group dialogue and communication as mechanisms for communal decision-making and consensus-building. In traditional societies, people see themselves as integral parts of a larger whole, leading to a strong sense of responsibility towards their community's wellbeing. Traditional and indigenous belief systems often incorporate holistic worldviews that view humans, nature, and the spiritual realm as interconnected, with dialogue as a means to maintain this delicate balance.

Many indigenous spiritual traditions' circle gatherings include rituals and ceremonies which are reflected in spiritual and religious traditions worldwide. Spiritual groups use group dialogue for community cohesion and personal growth but also for sharing interpretations and experiences of spiritual teachings, for increasing insight and deepening understanding, creating a sense of shared wisdom. Seekers come together to engage in dialogue, meditation, prayer, chanting, and to discuss spiritual teachings, struggles, doubts, and achievements. Increasing support and encouragement in shared vulnerability fosters empathy, compassion and a sense of identity and belonging among peers; participants develop deep bonds and a sense of collective identity. Elders may guide the group in self-inquiry and the exploration of an ultimate reality, transmitting spiritual teachings, practices, and rituals from one generation to another. Through storytelling, discussions and debates, elders pass down their wisdom to younger members, ensuring the continuity of the tradition. This transmission of tradition helps preserve cultural heritage and spiritual knowledge and increases wisdom and compassion. In Buddhism, these are known as Dharma talks; in Sufism, Suhbas; in Hinduism, Satsang. In Quakerism, with its emphasis on direct spiritual experience and communal discernment, meetings are held for worship where members gather in silence to wait upon the Inner Light or the presence of God. Participants may feel moved to share messages or lead the group in vocal prayer or hymns, fostering a sense of spiritual communion and collective discernment.

EAST AND WEST DIALOGUES

Group dialogue approaches can vary significantly between Eastern and Western philosophies due to differences in their underlying principles, values, and cultural contexts. Eastern philosophies such as Buddhism, Confucianism, and Taoism often emphasise interconnectedness, harmony, and the idea that individuals are part of a larger whole. They focus on inner transformation. Western philosophies, including those from ancient Greece to modern Western thought, tend to prioritise individualism, reason, and critical thinking. The emphasis is often on personal autonomy and individual rights.

Eastern group dialogue approaches often revolve around practices like meditation, mindfulness, and non-violent communication. These approaches encourage individuals to listen deeply, cultivate empathy, and seek harmony within the group. Dialogues may aim at reaching a collective understanding rather than proving individual points. Eastern philosophies often see the self as interconnected with others and the environment. Dialogues in this context may focus on transcending the ego and recognising the shared humanity in all participants. Eastern approaches often prioritise conflict transformation through understanding and empathy. Dialogue participants seek common ground and aim for win-win solutions. Conflict is seen as an opportunity for growth and understanding. Eastern group dialogues can include elements of spiritual inquiry and self-discovery. Questions may revolve around the nature of consciousness, suffering, and the pursuit of inner peace.

Western group dialogue approaches have developed within the context of Western intellectual traditions and have been influenced by the Enlightenment, classical philosophy, and modern thought. Western philosophies tend to emphasise the uniqueness of individuals, so group dialogue approaches may emphasise debate, structured discussions, argumentation, the presentation of evidence, critical thinking, and the exchange of ideas. Individuals assert their viewpoints and defend their positions, sometimes leading to competition rather than harmony. The goal is often to arrive at a rational consensus or resolution. Western group dialogues tend to centre on rational inquiry into topics such as ethics, politics, and epistemology. Participants often use logic and evidence to support their arguments.

It's important to note that these distinctions are generalisations, and there can be significant variation within each tradition and overlap between them, especially in today's globalised world where diverse philosophical perspectives often interact and influence one another.

DIALOGUE IN PRACTICE

Dialogue differs from other modes of communication such as discussion, which offers a more open format and is less rigid than debate. Debate is a structured exchange between two opposing sides, each arguing for or against a specific issue and while it can be useful for making definitive decisions, it also reinforces adversarial thinking, a common feature of Western culture. A monologue is a one-way communication, such as in storytelling or giving a presentation. The confusion around the word dialogue is many people think dialogue is 'two' and we occasionally hear 'trialogue' and even *quadrologue*.

Whether we view Dialogue from a Western philosophical lens of Enaction or an Eastern lens of Interbeing it doesn't matter; as a practice, Dialogue is meaning-making, together. Dialogue moves us from fragmentation to wholeness – through full participation and inclusiveness. A deep sense of belonging, underpinned by a profound dialogic ethos of unity, represented by each member being 'part of the whole' (circle), is crucial for maintaining the cohesiveness of a community; maintaining a strong support network and ultimately, self-realisation. Through dialogue, we may seek to understand our place in the cosmos, fostering a profound sense of self, spirituality and harmony with the world around us; not only ensuring the survival of cultural knowledge but also strengthening intergenerational bonds through new and meaningful ways of communication.

In the face of cultural erosion and assimilation, communities use group dialogue and communication as tools to enhance a way of being. Dialogues enable us to make sense together, spiritually advance, create shared meaning, reconnect with our roots, relearn traditional practices, and both revive and create new languages. This holistic sense of belonging, underpinned by a sound dialogic ethos, is crucial for maintaining the cohesiveness of a community and maintaining a strong support network. By doing so, we not only preserve our cultural heritage and enhance human endeavour through mutual enquiry but also promote a sense of meaning, fulfilment, identity and pride.

In an increasingly individualistic and fragmented society, group dialogues provide a space for meaningful connection and authentic communication, offering an antidote to the loneliness and isolation prevalent in modern life, and fostering a sense of belonging and mutual support. In a world increasingly characterised by cultural diversity, group dialogues contribute to cross-cultural understanding and appreciation, with some outstanding examples covered later on in this book.

I once facilitated a large dialogue circle of 65 people at The Beshara School in Scotland. The school is an example of how the 'sacred principles' of interconnectedness, taught in universities and via the Ibn Arabi Society in Oxford, can be integrated via 'conversation', applied wisdom and metaphysics into the wider world. The Beshara Trust states:

> The object for which the Trust is established is the advancement of education in the consideration of the basic unity of all religions, in particular by the provision of courses to provide an understanding of the relationship of man to the universe, the earth, the environment and the society he lives in, to Reality and to God.
>
> *(Beshara Trust, 2022, para 1)*

Recognising the wisdom embedded in our spiritual traditions can inspire us to cultivate similar practices in our societies, fostering greater harmony, empathy, and unity among all people, for example, using group dialogue and communication as a means of resolving conflicts.

By bringing together people from different backgrounds and traditions, dialogues promote empathy, tolerance, respect for diversity, and offer individuals opportunities for personal growth and self-discovery. Through reflective listening, constructive feedback, and open dialogue, participants can explore their beliefs, values, and aspirations, leading to greater self-awareness and fulfilment. For people involved in social justice, politics and activism, dialogues can be powerful tools, bringing together like-minded individuals to discuss pressing issues, share experiences, and strategise for change, catalysing collective action and fostering solidarity.

So by now we have established what Dialogue is – it involves a group of people engaging in a free-flowing conversation where they suspend their assumptions, listen deeply, hold maximum respect for themselves, each other and the process, and speak authentically. Group cohesion is really important and the goals are to foster mutual understanding, uncover collective meaning, and enable shared insights to emerge.

Dialogue is not only a method for discussing abstract or philosophical topics but can also be applied to various fields, including education, problem-solving, conflict resolution, and team building. By fostering an environment of open, empathetic, and non-judgmental communication, it encourages participants to explore their own thinking and collectively deepen their understanding of complex issues, leading to personal and collective growth and transformation.

Dialogue is not:

- Two people or groups talking in a film, play, on a bus or anywhere else
- Personal therapy[1]
- Supervision space (bringing in cases)
- A support group
- A personal development group[2]
- Cross conversations that are not relevant to the whole group
- Agenda driven.

REFERENCES

Beshara Trust. (2022). About the Beshara Trust. Retrieved from https://beshara.org/about-beshara-trust-21/
Bohm, D. (1980). *Wholeness and the Implicate Order*. Routledge & Kegan Paul.
Bohm, D. (1996). *On Dialogue*. Routledge Classics.
Center for Adaptive Stress. (2022). About the Evolutionary Stress Framework. Retrieved from https://ndstress.wordpress.com/about-the-esf/
Dunbar, R. & Shultz, S. (2007) Evolution of the social brain. *Science*, 317, 1344–1347. http://dx.doi:10.1126/science.1145463
Hogenkamp, L. (2018). Is autism a stress adaptation of neurodivergent neurotypes? Retrieved from https://peripheralmindsofautism.com/2018/04/17/is-autism-a-stress-adaptation/
Isaacs, W. N. (1996). The process and potential of dialogue in social change. *Educational Technology*, 36(1), 20–30.
Online Etymology Dictionary. (n.d.). Dialogue. Retrieved from www.etymonline.com/search?q=dialogue&utm_campaign=sd&utm_medium=serp&utm_source=ds_search

---

1 Although there are therapeutic benefits, and people may experience this and feel supported, the purpose of dialogue is not to provide personal therapy, supervision or support.
2 It is not a personal development group and it does not involve cross conversations that are not relevant to the whole group.

CHAPTER 4

Bringing together autism and Dialogue

Dialogue gives a voice to mechanisms that were previously difficult to be articulated or understood. In Dialogue, everyone's differences and uniqueness arise and if autism is to be explored universally this way, it needs a robust framework; a dynamic structure to ongoing, multi-level communications. The setting, the participants and the systems at play might contain varying elements of the psychodynamic, scientific, psychological, sociological, philosophical, metaphysical, and spiritual, and to be truly effective, it must also be completely practical. The power of dialogue is in acceptance and coming to terms with everything that's present and manifesting in that exact situation.

Dialogue works towards a flowing, holistic character of language, this correlates with the experience of autism. While accounting for and measuring all the variables that a Dialogue encounters is impossible, immersion in these settings is useful for improving affect, increasing self-compassion and reducing perceived stress for participants, both autistic and non-autistic. We know this from a lot of anecdotal and some qualitative evidence and evaluations.

Picture a calm room, a circle of around 12 people sitting on comfortable chairs with a gap between each person. After the facilitators provide some preliminary housekeeping (timing, breaks, location of toilets etc.), the session might begin with a few minutes guided relaxation and then a bit of a talk from the facilitators. Then the whole group decides on some ground rules. There are usually two facilitators; a lead and a support. Sessions need to last at least two to three hours and a series of at least six weekly or fortnightly sessions. Sometimes they can go on for up to six hours. For a suggested outline for running community sessions, see Appendix 1.

Dialogue, like nature, is a regenerative feedback system; it promotes unity of thinking. Allison Leigh Holt describes this in the excellent paper 'The Conversation: Feedback Structures, Ways of Knowing, and Neurodivergence' (Holt, 2019).

All living beings participate in a vast, astounding feedback system comprised of a community of feedback systems. This perceiving-sensing, adjusting-processing, and responding-exchanging is communication, beyond language; between humans and the not-quite-fixed world of all things that exist, with or without categorization, and between those things themselves. Meaningful communication between human and non-human species is contingent upon first reconsidering our understanding of human consciousness and cognition.

In terms of autism, this relative 'not-quite-fixed world … with or without categorization' can be compared to Gestalt Perception (Bogdashina, 2022) – with difficulty in filtering out 'information' (or indeed, defining information in the first place. Autism then, might be understood as a different way of accessing or processing Bohm's Implicate Order. It is highly likely that autistic individuals 'perceive or experience reality' in a manner that diverges from the neurotypical experience, possibly sensing connections or details that others do not. So, is it possible autistics are more attuned to the nuances of how 'things' relate to each other within a given environment?

Erin Manning (2018) argues that this form of awareness is fundamental to all perception – what we perceive is an interconnected ecology before subject or object. From this perspective, Manning suggests we consider an ecological politics that prioritises movement and relationships over fixed categories, which can be polarising (such as neurotypical versus neurodivergent, or human versus nonhuman or even teacher versus student).

There are further well-known implications of brain filtering in Autism, which produce issues, for example, sensory modulation – when the brain isn't filtering out enough information and there is simply too much information for the brain to process, it tries to pay attention to everything and sensory overload may occur, resulting in meltdown or shutdown – responses of the nervous system. Perhaps this is because modern environments, which aim to cater for the maximum number of people, are generally fragmented. Think of a supermarket with thousands of products, crowds, bright lights, smells, auditory reverb, constantly changing temperatures and then outside negotiating car parks and busy streets.

In Dialogue as a praxis, action and thinking work dialectically so it's always dynamic, in that dialogue transforms the world in which the practice is carried out. Dialogue must always be pragmatic and participants should readily access, and relate to, the wider context for processing and assimilation to keep the content and topics socially relevant. They must bring authentic, real-world concerns and perceptions. To attend to a harmonious, slower-paced, circle-shaped conversational gathering, with predictability and structure, enhances and replenishes the sense of unity – in oneself and one's environment, be that in situ or wider definitions including family, friends, school, work etc. Given the incompatibility of our modern environments, it's no wonder many autistics claim that recovery is the main benefit at the start of attending Dialogues.

Manning (2018) invites us to explore what it would mean to adopt an ecological politics of collective individuation through language – which supports Bohm's (1980) rheo-mode of (flowing) language (with emphasis on the verb instead of the noun).

Bohm's idea that reality is not strictly linear could align with the autistic experience of non-linear thinking, time, sensory processing and cognition, which sometimes appears more fragmented or nonlinear compared to the less flexible 'neurotypical' mind. This could provide insights into why autistics might struggle with, or excel in certain tasks, depending on their alignment with the Implicate Order's deeper patterns. Essentially Bohm's 'Holism' Dialogue approach inspires us towards more inclusive education, social policies and environments, by promoting holistic strategies that help neurodivergent people integrate their perspectives. The term 'autism friendly' has some way to go.

Because of the slipperiness of the autism construct, nowadays I simply say 'I was told I meet the criteria'. My Gestalt therapist didn't seem to think Asperger's was at all relevant to my healing process – fair enough! Later, as I sat in on the local Autism Partnership Board and Strategy and Training subgroups, the different politically correct attempts to address autism left me feeling rather confused and objectified. Studying autism at postgraduate level helped provide some background to this mysterious phenomenon, and in a coaching and mentoring course, I learned firsthand of the lack of neurodiversity-aware approaches to coaching, writing a case study for this in the book *Ethical Case Studies for Coach Development and Practice: A Coach's Companion* (Drury, 2023).

Around the same time, the idea for Autism Dialogues occurred to me. Addressing the unknown about both autism and the self simultaneously is where the original spirit for Autism Dialogue resides. It seemed simple to me that in safe and conducive micro-communities, I and others like me might be able to 'drop the mask', recover and relax (although I've explored the problems with masking as a concept in this book elsewhere). Sometimes in our societies, masking (especially for autistic people where there are involuntary conforming tendencies) makes life less enjoyable and complicated and, in unforgiving environments, it happens a lot. Recovery seemed to be the first stage in the process of dialogue for us so-called autistic people and there had to be so-called non-autistic people in the room. In creating these encounters, I had to somehow mirror the societal problem, with ethics and safety. 'ADA' started as being about what happens when autistic and non-autistic people come together, for a safely challenging, collective synergy. Recovery, understanding, improved wellbeing and community cohesion through exploring and refining our communication, were the aspects of life we could all understand and begin to work with. I don't think the approach has shifted much since these initial aims.

At a conference, I heard an autism researcher present a talk about a large project they were involved in, which included dealing with two essential elements: Ontology (relating to the question 'who am I?') and Epistemology ('what do I know?'). Being from a well-funded and forward-thinking academic research group, they concluded that they couldn't understand why, for years they hadn't previously seen the crucial place of these two questions when studying autism. In Dialogue, these questions are fundamental.

Ask yourself now: Who am I? What do I know?

Bohm and many others have claimed communication in our societies is in crisis, and by exploring language, meaning and communication in the autism context, we take humble steps into the unknown together, to open up new space for potential and generative dialogue.

For me, Dialogue is dropping down into the heart. Dialogue is not agenda-driven, debate, politics, spiritual, a platform for airing views, silent consensus, intervention or therapy. But it may contain elements of all of these and it is for us to examine them together – safely … if and when they arise. It is, quite simply, Dialogue.

Do we purposefully avoid tension and conflict? Not at all, but with no agenda, some of the typical tensions that might arise with language limitations are far less likely. Emotions can and do run high but it is amazing to witness how the collective rallies round to genuinely support the individual in a moment of need or overwhelming breakthrough. In an exercise I spontaneously brought into one session, I suggested for a moment that everyone listen to the sounds in the room.

Try it yourself now. Now relax and consider the following: What if the reason you are here is not the reason you thought you were here? Think about that for a moment.

This is how, in our dialogue circles, we gently open up potential, by accepting the unknown and unknowable and that allows trust to grow.

THE IMPORTANCE OF MINDFUL AWARENESS

Using self-focus and meditation since my youth, I've helped myself to combat much of the sensory and social insensitivities of the world; I now teach others to do the same in Mindfulness for Autism workshops. Like many, I may come across as confident but to my detriment, often the more nervous I am, the more confident I appear; I used to be extremely controlling but have learned to manage this as well, through dialogue among other things. Meditation has been a major way of grounding, and I couldn't do without it. I'm deeply concerned with many things and overall what I'm doing here in this body, world and life, and why shouldn't I be? Deep reflection on the presence and the workings of the body and mind is an invaluable pastime. Awareness and techniques to increase it are fundamental to the practice of Dialogue. I try to work with the non-dual aspects of this life of autism, dismantling and exploring the 'us and them', me and you, autistic, non-autistic, neurodivergent and neurotypical, me and it, this 'I've got it' or 'it's got me' or 'I'm in this movement not that one'…me and my autism. I'm here and inside each of us there's an untouched 'is-ness', and our experiences are as much a part of us as we are them.

However, to avoid getting too abstract, fighting for justice and rights in our society is what the marginalised need to do, but as Nick Hodge (2017, p. 14) put it, 'rights are only activated if the dominant group recognises first the humanity of those made marginal and then acknowledges its corresponding duties to protect these rights'. Identifying as autistic is a step on the journey. Examining autism from the perspective of an integrated whole enters the realms of metaphysics, and approaching notions of 'the self' in the English language, becomes less tenable. I sympathise with Dr Olga Bogdashina who has been criticised for being too broad in her approach to autism, which covers a very broad range of sciences. In another case of language-shifting, 'environmental consciousness' takes on other meanings when we consider that autism is an ecology in a social environment and the personal impact we all have on each other in our shared spaces.

EXPERIENCES IN EARLY DIALOGUE SESSIONS

In an Autism Dialogue session, no one has to speak. Listening is one of the four practices and we must also value silent recovery. We avoid placing undue attention on participants and autistic people should be supported to use non-normative modes of communication, even telepathy if that is their chosen way. A human gift is that your flow of thought is known only to you, even in a total change of heart.

In our early dialogues, we decided to address a common duality; that of autistic and the non-autistic. We thought about it and wrangled with it together and then the non-autistic people went away and we ran three sessions with just autistic people, and then all came back together for a final three hour session. By assembling our micro-society, dismantling and reassembling it, we could interrogate and soften the boundaries. Author and researcher Nick Chown states, 'the ontological status of both the autistic and non-autistic neurotypes is partly dependent upon the nature of the society. We might want to say that the ontological status is socially constructed to this extent' (Chown, 2014, p. 1675). From within this delightful perspective, in a Dialogue session, we are co-creating our own society with meaning-making and everything else.

There should be more spaces in society to enable its own interrogation of our assumptions of humanness and normalcy, culture and notions of identity. Interestingly, there is growing evidence that autistic people understand each other in specific ways (Heasman & Gillespie, 2018; Crompton et al., 2020) – and we can look forward to further developments in that area and explore them in our activities. By creating our intersubjective environments, the autism community can go beyond a culture of fear and blame to one of familiarity and collective power on a more proactive ground.

Autism doesn't distinguish between people or types and nor should Dialogue, and everyone should be welcome to participate. If participants can understand the aims, intentions and practices (and here is one of the challenges) then there is participation and infinite potential – at the microcosmic level with change at the macrocosmic. Challenges arise though; for example, one may ask, what can we do about unheard voices – those who aren't in the room for whatever reason? This is a question we've asked many times and it has at times been very uncomfortable. Who are we to speak on anyone's behalf? I once read in an academic paper, the researchers' claim of 'capturing voices of those who do not speak'. It made me want to run away!

Increasingly elaborate scientific research into this thing we simply call autism, can detract us from the fact that people need supporting, enabling, empowering and they, we, need help to do this now. And it makes sense the more of a collective we all are, the more we can move towards what we all want out of life. National spending priority should be placed on applied research to help people living with neurological differences, instead of on basic genetic, biological and medical research.

The Autism Dialogue Approach is an inclusive, strengths-based approach incorporating cross-neurotype and cross-cultural perspectives. It is systems-sensitive in that it allows multiple perspectives to co-exist. It provides a range of obvious benefits for autistic people, such as a safe micro-community environment that mirrors society. It is participatory meaning-making in action. The efficacy and effectiveness of cross-neurotype intersubjectivity and within-interaction analysis is a viable methodology serving as its own research-to-practice ecosystem and can challenge the typical knowledge-transfer orthodoxy.

Studying autism in higher education was problematic. Experimental research designs in the autism education field are based on a 'knowledge-transfer' model of evidence-based practice, in which research is conducted by researchers, and is then transferred to practitioners to enable them to implement evidence-based interventions. While these research designs contribute important knowledge, they lead to a gap between what the research evidence may prescribe and what happens in practice, with a concomitant disparity between the priorities of researchers and practitioners (Guldberg et al., 2017). I increasingly hear from people that 'the whole education system needs overhauling'. We can point the blame at education or any one area of a system, but it's like the Zen master who, testing his student, asked him, 'Where is the moon?' When the student pointed up behind the master, the finger was abruptly chopped off. According to Zen, the moon is already in your head.

Bohm knew that when we lose authenticity and openness to the fact that everything is ultimately part of the whole, things go very wrong. Dialogue is already implicitly political and rife with elements of social justice, because it gathers and transmits influences, energy and narratives with varying levels of trust, listening, respect and judgement from authentic human thinking and voices. Our fundamental values, perpetually spread in communication, gather and are harnessed in Dialogue, to explore, dissect and reshuffle to disrupt and trouble the status quo with new power. Dialogue does this not by design, but simply because that's what happens; the universe and all its elements – people, animals, insects, plants and rocks – are inherently good. People walk away from Dialogue revitalised and with renewed trust in people and their world and the world. The process of extrication from old, stuck systems can at first be problematic for the autistic individual who, once intensely themselves as a hyper-sensitive, self-protecting bundle of nerves, has their very identity challenged in a safe, empowering new container. Setting out as the first Autism

Dialogue Facilitator, I felt all sorts of strange dynamics, including the possibility that I was perpetuating the myths of autism.

Being hyper-empathetic, studying one's relationship with others opens one up further, which requires self-care. Relational tension within oneself, the spectrum of family, friends, community, nature, the universe and God, or the sacred, are often all at stake in Dialogue. On a practical level, the social activist in a Dialogue might invite the exploring of a fairer society, with rights and education for all and use words like belonging, diversity and inclusion. Using 'I' statements is encouraged however – fight for your right when it's threatened, but make sure you truly know that right is yours to begin with. In a Dialogue, this can be examined and you might find that what's reflected back at you is that we also have a right to not have rights – the right to be nothing. Human belonging is fundamental to life, but we can't really belong, or promote belonging, if we don't know who we are or where or how we are situated – or meant to be – to begin with. Otherwise, the world would be a very different place. And a dialogue facilitator has to be on everyone's side.

Dialogue as advocated by Bohm and colleagues, allows multiple perspectives to co-exist in the same space of enquiry and understanding, slowing down normative modes of interaction into more of an evolving, unified flow. Active participation is generated and people develop an open mindset, learning to genuinely embrace diversity and respectfully engage with a range of viewpoints. Through transformational learning with each other, everyone develops curiosity and connects in deep and powerful ways. This is the basis of community, where creativity, love and expression of beauty are the supreme guiding principles. In co-creative Dialogue, thought and language are the paints and brushes and the space between is the canvas.

As an example, in educational Autism Dialogues, through direct encounters with those who are different, students might be empowered to overcome prejudice and armoured against those whose narrative seeks to divide. They will acquire a range of skills as their neuro-differences are engaged sensitively and respectfully, while developing greater confidence and self-esteem.

Younger people (and in many cases older, creative people) not only understand things through words like all of us but also invent words and are the meaning-makers of words. At the core of Dialogue is participatory meaning-making and sense-creating, which is also a signifier of pure, conscious awareness. A project which aims to uncover inherent social dilemmas and issues from the autistic perspective creates, generates or gives rise to hidden tensions, and participants will try to work with these dilemmas, and in seeing them, they are somehow, in a mysterious yet pragmatic way, resolved. Autism Dialogue is relentless and rigorous in self-enquiry. When it works well and the whole group hovers on the edge of meaning, it can be felt as an impersonal *koinonia* – a Greek word meaning impersonal fellowship. It's a rare, intimate and transcendent experience. Dialogue is consciously co-creating together. Dialogue is a name for the ultimate divine principle, as it is the creativity of the Absolute, and at the heart of that creativity is communication and communion. Mikhail Bakhtin referred to our true inter-relating as the sacred space: 'The single adequate form for verbally expressing authentic human life is the open-ended dialogue. Life by its very nature is dialogic' (Bakhtin, 1984 [1929], p. 293).

Of course, the Autism Dialogue Approach isn't for everyone, but if you're still interested, you'll need to learn and embody some basic understanding and principles.

REFERENCES

Bakhtin, M. (1984 [1929]). *Problems of Dostoevsky's Poetics*. Trans. C. Emerson. University of Minnesota Press.

Bogdashina, O. (2022). The role of sensory perceptual differences in autism: the 'Intense World Syndrome' and other sensory theories. Retrieved from www.olgabogdashina.com/post/the-role-of-sensory-perceptual-differences-in-autism

Bohm, D. (1980). *Wholeness and the Implicate Order.* Routledge & Kegan Paul.

Chown, N. P. (2014). More on the ontological status of autism and double empathy. Disability & Society 29(10), 1672–1676. http://dx.doi.org/10.1080/09687599.2014.949625

Crompton, C. J., Ropar, D., Evans-Williams, C. V., Flynn, E. G. & Fletcher-Watson, S. (2020). Autistic peer-to-peer information transfer is highly effective. Autism, 24(7), 1704–1712. https://doi.org/10.1177/1362361320919286

Drury, J. (2023). Case study 35: coaching in the neurodivergent landscape. In W. Smith, E. Hirsch Pontes, D. Magadlele & D. Clutterbuck (eds), *Ethical Case Studies for Coach Development and Practice. A Coach's Companion* (pp 180–183). Routledge.

Guldberg, K., Parsons, S., Porayska-Pomsta, K. & Keay-Bright, W. (2017). Challenging the knowledge-transfer orthodoxy: knowledge co-construction in technology-enhanced learning for children with autism. British Educational Research Journal, 43(2), 394–413. https://doi.org/10.1002/berj.3275

Heasman, B. & Gillespie, A. (2018). Perspective-taking is two-sided: misunderstandings between people with Asperger's syndrome and their family members. Autism, 22(6), 740–750. https://doi.org/10.1177/1362361317708287

Hodge, N. (2017). Developing the rights approach for autism. Paper presented at Autism Centre Professorial Inaugural Presentation, Sheffield, UK, 14 March.

Holt, A. (2019). The conversation: feedback structures, ways of knowing, and neurodivergence. Public, 30(59), 104–112. https://doi.org/10.1386/public.30.59.104_1

Manning, E. (2018). Histories of violence: neurodiversity and the policing of the norm. Retrieved from https://lareviewofbooks.org/article/histories-of-violence-neurodiversity-and-the-policing-of-the-norm

PART II

Communities of meaning-making

CHAPTER 5

Introduction to Dialogue in autism contexts

....

THE KEY PRINCIPLES AND AIMS OF AUTISM DIALOGUE

The Autism Dialogue Approach (ADA) is a whole-system, psychosocial framework that facilitates participatory, generative dialogue, using a simple yet powerful set of practices with skilled facilitation. Building mainly on what has been gleaned from my experience and understanding of Bohm (or Bohmian) Dialogue, I applied a new iteration of the framework to provide safe, confidential, and non-judgmental environments for people to explore autism, including me. The remit went along the lines of 'all who are impacted by misunderstandings and exclusion can come together to foster improved relationships, share experiences and develop common understanding and acceptance, for better lives, work and vocations'. Note that I said 'all who are impacted', meaning exactly that – and 'impacted' can be interpreted positively.

Not formulating a model was easy – I always intuitively went by what William Isaacs says:

> Because the nature of Dialogue is exploratory, its meaning and its methods continue to unfold. No firm rules can be laid down for conducting a Dialogue because its essence is learning – not as the result of consuming a body of information or doctrine imparted by an authority, not of a means of examining a particular theory or program, rather as part of an unfolding process of creative participation between peers.
>
> *(Isaacs, 1999)*

I did set one benchmark though, after some strong views from certain members of a group – that is that if someone were autistic, they would need to be able to identify as such, to the group, and not intentionally come to sit on the fence about whether they were autistic or not. This was to preserve integrity for those who ascribe to being autistic (and the identity itself), to subtly invite a sense of assertiveness into their doubt and bring this attitude to support the fold. Wondering if you were autistic once you were in the group was different. However, this was just one specific piece of contracting and clearly, there can be spaces where people can intentionally set out to explore their autistic-ness, and you may wish to explore that in your own way. During one series at the Sheffield Quaker Meeting House, Dr. Dinah Murray was quite vocal to me about there being no researchers present, to avoid what she called 'fishbowling' and I had the unenviable task of letting a local academic know they were no longer welcome in the group.

ADA is a unique, novel approach, inspired and informed by a variety of sources including experiences of autism and neurodivergence, a wide range of established dialogic modalities, Western and Eastern philosophies, sociological theory, neuroscience and a broad range of coaching philosophies and approaches, continually adapted (and co-designed by participants) for suitability in the fields of human interpersonal development and inclusion issues. With a set of easily learned practices described below, participants work to diminish their own fragmented thinking to co-create cohesive wholeness in the self, their organisation and the community. ADA directly addresses fragmentation by seeing the individual person, group and external society as a single entity. Knowledge transfer and learning is always relevant, being delivered by, and to those who are present in safe and confidential settings. Shared information, experiences, thinking and genuine feelings can be exchanged in a real-world, safe and confidential neurodiverse microcommunity. Participants are encouraged to 'come as yourself' and feel safe to come and go as they please without being judged. Co-produced reports were a conduit for sharing findings and taking better decisive action towards shared and newly aligned goals.

EXPLICIT AIMS

In summary, the Autism Dialogue Approach aims to:

- Shift mainstream perceptions, replace negative, deficit-based stereotypes and show that all society benefits from the incorporation of *neurominorities*.
- Raise the status of neurodivergent/autistic people and those impacted, especially families and organisations.
- Support and benefit neurodivergent/autistic people and those impacted, especially families.
- Improve, enhance and strengthen the inclusion of neurodivergent people's access to essential services and in the workplace where typically, learning is challenging and impacted by the environment.
- Release into society what is believed to be huge untapped potential in neurodivergent/autistic minds.
- Improve cohesion of the autism communities through raising of understanding, awareness and acceptance of autism.
- Negate the impact of challenging environments, reduce anxiety and stress, help reduce the frequency and intensity of meltdowns, shutdowns and overloads and improve overall wellbeing and quality of life for autistic people.

THE FOUR PRACTICES

Dialogue is a method that requires some basic understanding, but is easy to learn because it has its roots in ancestral story-sharing, which we all used to do when we lived in villages and more traditional communities. There has evolved a set of easily learned skills that help to guide a group into an aligned way of thinking together. The four dialogic practices enhance our ability to connect with others, and, when applied well, they can enhance our collective sense-making and our ability to participate on a deeper level. Dialogue seeks to transform both how we think and how we reflect on our thinking. This change happens collectively as a large group engages in conversation within a circle. It is achieved through four core practices – listening, respecting, suspending and voicing. These four practices were developed by William Isaacs (1999), drawing on four key principles that Bohm suggested as fundamental to the structure of the world, including the neurology of thought.

They are in fact, the elements of any good conversation. Authentic conversation is about speaking honestly and vulnerably, while suspension of assumptions challenges us to remain open-minded and curious. Deep listening enables us to engage with others empathetically and respectfully, fostering trust and understanding in our interactions.

1. Authentic voice

Authenticity lies at the heart of meaningful communication. When we speak with our authentic voice, we share our thoughts, feelings, and experiences genuinely and transparently. This practice encourages us to be honest and vulnerable, to express ourselves without fear of judgement or rejection. By speaking from the heart, we create an environment of trust and openness, inviting others to do the same. Authentic voice fosters genuine connections, allowing us to relate to one another on a deeper, more personal level. Sensitive conversation also requires a commitment to authenticity – the courage to speak our truth with honesty and integrity, even when it's uncomfortable or difficult.

Authenticity is not just about speaking our truth; it's also about honouring the truth of others. It's about recognising that everyone has their own unique perspective, their own truth to share, and their own story to tell. When we approach conversation with an open mind and a willingness to learn from others, we create space for diverse voices and experiences to be heard and respected.

2. Listening

Deep listening goes beyond simply hearing the words that are spoken; it involves fully engaging with the speaker on a deeper level. Deep listening involves being present in the moment, giving the speaker our full attention, and empathetically tuning into their thoughts and feelings. By listening deeply, we demonstrate respect and validation for the speaker's experiences, fostering trust and empathy in the conversation.

Listening is a skill that is as rare as it is valuable in today's fast-paced world, where distractions abound and attention spans are dwindling. This practice requires us to pay attention not only to what is being said but also to their body language, tone of voice, emotional cues and felt energy fluctuations. It means setting aside our own agenda and ego, giving the speaker our undivided attention, validating their feelings and experiences, and responding authentically with empathy and respect. Yet, it is precisely in its precious rarity that its power lies, as when we truly listen to one another – without judgement, without interruption, without distraction – we create a space where people feel seen, heard, and valued. And in this space, meaningful connections can flourish, against all odds.

3. Respect

Respect is the foundation of meaningful communication. It involves treating others with dignity, empathy and consideration, regardless of differences or disagreements. This practice requires us to honour each person's unique perspective, value their experiences and contributions, and engage with them in a spirit of mutual respect. Respectful communication creates an environment of trust and safety, where all voices are heard and valued. The collective, subtly changing process is respected too – and is based on 'coherence,'; involving seeing commonality in differences without seeking agreement. Respect in groups allows polarities to coexist without rushing to resolve them.

It fosters empathy and understanding, allowing for constructive dialogue, meaningful connections and new insight to flourish.

4. Suspension

We all carry a set of assumptions, beliefs, and biases that shape our perceptions of the world. However, these assumptions can often lead to misunderstandings and conflicts in communication. The practice of suspending assumptions involves setting aside our preconceived notions and approaching each conversation with an open mind. It requires us to challenge our own biases, to question our assumptions, and to remain curious and receptive to new ideas and perspectives. By suspending assumptions, we create space for genuine dialogue and mutual understanding, allowing for the exploration of diverse viewpoints and experiences.

Dialogue facilitator Jessica Ball (2024), in adding a number of further guidelines emphasises early participation, suggesting at the beginning of a dialogue the facilitator invites participants to read the guidelines together, each person reading one out loud, if desired. Ball also accommodates for visual thinking by the use of friendly pictorials, which can be seen on her website.

USING THE FOUR PRACTICES IN A GROUP

Awareness and practice of dialogue principles shape a group, and support a development approach that resonates with others naturally, as these principles may be inherently 'hard-wired' into us. Together, these practices create a framework for sensitive conversation, allowing us to build meaningful connections and cultivate empathy and compassion in all of our relationships. Being always mindful of them is good practice, and they should be introduced to a Dialogue programme cohort as early as possible, as part of preparatory material, with other basic guidance, to foster a welcoming spirit and reduce any pre-concerns. The practices are to be agreed upon, learned, followed, embodied and referred to throughout a programme. Remind yourself and your participants that they are a practice because the more you practise them, the better you will be at using them. It is likely that many people won't understand that there can be rules or even guidance to communicating effectively so it is also useful to invite people to relax and not overly focus on them, particularly at the beginning where it might take a few sessions to understand on a deep, embodied level. We all have a lot of unlearning to do.

Bringing the spirit of the four practices from the start of the process of organising Dialogue, we can also be attentive to sensitive human needs, slower reading of emails, clearer posters, show diagrams, photographs, video and instructions and information about the physical venue or virtual environment.

FURTHER CONSIDERATIONS AROUND SENSITIVE CONVERSATION

In addition to the four practices that emerged from Bohm and his contemporaries for general usage, several elements have arisen during our autism work, which build on the former principles: 'What is needed is a means by which we can slow down the process of thought in order to be able to observe it while it is actually occurring.' (Bohm, Factor & Garrett, 1991, para. 10).

In meaningful human connection, conversation (in the loosest sense) serves as a crucial thread, weaving together our experiences, emotions, and perspectives into complex mosaics. At its essence, sensitive communication is grounded in empathy – that human quality to recognise and resonate with the emotions and experiences of others, which entails stepping into someone else's perspective, viewing the world through their lens, and responding with warmth and understanding. In a world marked by diversity and divergent opinions, empathy acts as a unifying force, enabling us to discover commonalities and forge meaningful bonds.

For autistic people, who are socially sensitive and often embody hyper-empathy on a scale many can't imagine, engaging in conversation can present unique challenges and experiences. Sensitive conversation takes on added significance for those with extremely heightened sensitivity to the emotions and nuances conveyed through language and dynamics of environment. Hyper-empathy can make navigating social interactions particularly intense, as autistics feel deeply impacted by the emotions of others, often to the point of overwhelm. Sensitive conversation from the autistic perspective involves not only understanding the spoken words of another but also deciphering the subtleties of tone, body language, social cues and relentless neuro-normative narratives and expectations of normalcy. There may be a requirement for a profound awareness of the emotional landscape of a conversation, often necessitating careful interpretation and processing of social signals coming from a person of the predominant neurotype and the fluctuations and dynamics of intersecting identities. Consider, for example, the difficulties an autistic person might face who hasn't used the internet for a while and upon entering a 'support group' is faced with a barrage of new terminologies which aim for a more inclusive society. In effect, the person is excluded who isn't 'up to date' with the latest identity language nuances. I've met several autistic people who've felt very confused by the growing emphasis on gender pronouns, for example, and preferred not to speak or even attend social gatherings for fear of 'getting it wrong'. Identity-affirming practices, while aiming for inclusion, aren't something all autistic people may understand, which can lead to exclusion.

Sensitive conversation requires a commitment to inclusivity – the recognition that everyone deserves to have their voice heard, regardless of their background, identity, or perspective. It's about creating space for marginalised voices, amplifying stories and experiences, and challenging the systems of power and privilege that silence them. When we approach conversation with a commitment to inclusivity, we create a more equitable and just society, where everyone has the opportunity to participate fully and authentically.

Empathy holds a significant role in the intricate dance of sensitive conversation for autistic people, who strive to bridge emotional gaps with others. Yet, this heightened empathy can become a double-edged sword, blurring the lines between one's own emotions and those of others. When the weight of expectation is upon the autistic person to 'learn' non-autistic communication, instead of equal responsibility to learn each other's modes, something happens to the relational dynamic. The phenomenon is commonly known as the double empathy problem (Milton, 2012), and for the autistic, can lead to emotional overload or exhaustion, making navigating social interactions even more challenging. It's interesting that the double empathy problem, while popularly referring to that gap between autistic and non-autistic, will play out directly among autistic people too.

Inclusive conversation is in Dialogue; the mode through which we move from fragmentation to wholeness. From the autistic viewpoint, sensitive conversation entails a profound reverence for individual differences and neurodiversity. It requires recognising and cherishing the varied ways in which individuals communicate and perceive the world, all while acknowledging the necessity for accommodation and understanding. I often wonder how the double empathy theory is perhaps limited as our fragmented world seems to have an infinite empathy problem!

While navigating sensitive conversations, autistic individuals often resort to strategies such as explicit communication, script-based interactions, and structured frameworks. These methods serve to enhance comprehension and diminish ambiguity, possibly fostering smoother exchanges, but at their expense. Fostering a nurturing and inclusive environment that embraces neurodiversity can significantly enrich the authenticity and depth of conversation for all.

Ultimately, from the autistic perspective, sensitive conversation is a quest for genuine connection and comprehension, all while respecting the diverse experiences and sensitivities of each participant. It is through empathy, acceptance, and mutual respect that meaningful connections are forged, enriching the tapestry of human interaction for both autistic individuals and 'neurotypicals' alike and for that matter all neurotypes. Sensitive conversation is not just about the words we speak, but the connections we forge – the moments of understanding, empathy, and solidarity that bring us closer together as human beings. It's about recognising the power of our words to heal or to harm, to build bridges or to erect barriers, and choosing to use them wisely and compassionately. And in embracing the art of sensitive dialogue, we rediscover the true joy of simply being together – in all our diversity, complexity, and wonderful human messiness.

THE BENEFITS OF AN ADA PRACTICE

> Dialogue creates shared meaning, values and a sense of community that supports joint action and the creation of culture.
> *(Bohm, 1996, cited in Meunier & Landry, 2008, p. 466).*

Based on personal experience and much testimony from hundreds of participants, it's safe to conclude that participation in Dialogue has the following benefits:

- Reduction of psychological stress and anxiety.
- Empowerment and greater self-knowledge.
- Increase in familiarity and promote deeper awareness, respect and openness.
- Improvement to quality of life and wellbeing.
- A more neurodivergent leadership culture.
- Reduction of pressure on waiting lists/doctors, via social prescribing and signposting.
- Cross-community cohesion leading to improved understanding, openness and a more enriched society.

This book isn't a scientific treatise and I've already laid out its limitations. I haven't claimed to have created a dialogue model based on evidence. There hasn't yet been any scientific research conducted on anything called Autism Dialogue; the reasons for this may or may not unfold in an appropriate series of research Dialogues.

Autism and all other neurodivergent perspectives (including dyslexia, dyscalculia, ADHD, Tourette's etc.) and acquired neurodivergence (such as brain injury, blindness etc.) are a catalyst and focal point for refining human awareness. Dialogue aims to examine diversity together to raise consciousness and quality of life, which naturally means adopting a dialogic approach to one's life. Knowledge generated from within the work of ADA, as well as the principles and practices themselves, is transferable to any field, be it personal, educational or professional, being unconstrained by a particular definition or context.

REFERENCES

Ball, J. (2024). David Bohm and Bohm dialogue. Retrieved from www.creatingmeaning.club/david-bohm-dialogue

Bohm, D., Factor, D. & Garrett, P. (1991). Dialogue – a proposal. Retrieved from https://aofpd.org/library/public-resources/dialogue-a-proposal/

Isaacs, W. (1999). *Dialogue and the Art of Thinking Together.* Bantam Doubleday Dell.

Meunier, A. & Landry, A. (2008). *La recherche en éducation muséale: actions et perspectives.* Éditions MultiMondes.

Milton, D. E. (2012). On the ontological status of autism: the 'double empathy problem'. Disability and Society, 27(6), 883–887.

CHAPTER 6

Autism theories and common themes

This book is not 'about autism'. Over the years in speaking to hundreds of people, I've seen the definition of autism shift from a fixed label or category into a question and an opportunity – for exploring what it means to be a self, in a world that's otherwise quick to categorise what selfhood is.

So far, I've tried to establish that any *dialogic* approach to exploring autism and neurodiversity is not merely about understanding autism and neurodiversity, it is about exploring the nature of oneself IN the world in a radical, dynamic and generative way. It challenges the view that an individual person can be deficient or damaged without involving the complexity of fragmented systems and thought. I don't think this can be emphasised enough: The autistic experience is also a pathway to greater self-awareness and joy. With increased mutual understanding, autism itself can be a source of awakening.

In Dialogue groups, it's possible to alleviate the negative impacts and clinical aspects of what we call autism, by listening to and studying the experiences and lives of those themselves whom we call autistic. From the monotropic cave art of early humans to global anthropomorphic phenomena and today's fascinating autistic-led theory, the answers to the problems autism presents us with are, I believe, lying in the open. In this chapter I have also included some notes on how aspects of some of the main autism theories relate to – and can impact – dialogue within a group context.

Autism has attracted a rhetoric of tragedy, pervasive narratives of deficit and chaotic societal tendencies, which seek to divide and maintain mass confusion, leading to othering, loneliness, self-harm and suicide. To be clear, the answers to what we call autism aren't under the microscope of *big pharma*, reductive sciences and behavioural conformity programmes:

> The way dominant society has dealt with autism is in lock step with the conversation we have chosen with our environment. Both are aspects of a misguided order of interpretation that separates us from one another and from

natural systems. The empirical, siloed epistemological framework in which we operate is untenable and failing.

(Holt, 2019, p. 111)

The autistic experience as deficit and the image of a broken and bereft person can be transformed into a rare kind of human who, like the ever-sensitive canary in the coal mine, is only temporarily sick because of their environment, and needs only our collaboration (getting us all out of the mine to begin with) to bring them back to full shining, singing glory and ultimately released from the cage. Any cure for autism would be to bring that allegorical canary back from the poisonous gases of conditioning and conformity, deep in the mine of society.

Autism presents as an opportunity; it is the mirror we seek which, once allowed to reflect our own shortcomings, will consolidate our long, forgotten ways. A single male canary will typically be content to live alone and sing to its heart's content.

If societal at all, I approach *autos-ism* as a crisis of selfhood. Humans are too often in possession of such a low level of sense of self and meaning, that not enough contentment exists for life to be worth living. Autism is a social phenomenon. According to the Diagnostic Manual (DSM V) (American Psychiatric Association, 2013) Autistic people, characteristically, experience challenges with social skills, repetitive behaviours and speech and nonverbal communication. When viewed as a way of being, at the core of the neurodiversity paradigm, (which we'll cover in chapter 9), autism invites us to appreciate the rich diversity of human experience and cognition. It represents a distinct neurological and cognitive profile that is part of the natural spectrum of human diversity.

WHAT IS AUTISM?

Autism is from Latin *autismus*, from Ancient Greek *autós* ('self') and Latin *-ismus* ('-ism'), and first coined by Swiss psychiatrist Eugene Bleuler in 1911. '*Dia*' is from the Greek for 'apart' or 'between' and 'gnosis' is from the Greek for 'knowledge'. Diagnosis is learning what sets something apart from other things. Many people consider and receive an autism diagnosis without knowing the meaning and origin of the words. Knowing yourself is very helpful and empowering.

- *autos* = self
- *ism* = system/ideology
- *dia* = through
- *gnosis* = knowledge
- *logos/legein* = meaning

= self systemising through knowing and meanings.

So the general supposition is: Know yourself through systemising self-knowledge and meaning-making. The term 'autism diagnosis' can point to the healthy, natural and dynamic human pursuit of self-enquiry: The definition of autism, like the self, is a process; a continually evolving and self-creating construct. I've been creative in coming to this conclusion too.

With a sharp look at the origins of the term autism, Paul Harris (2000) describes how, to fit their own theories, Kanner (and later Piaget), bent Bleuler's hypothesis of autism being a characteristic of all human minds, stating:

> Today, we normally associate the term 'autistic' with the developmental pathology first identified by Kanner (1943). Kanner borrowed Bleuler's terminology because the children that he had observed displayed a withdrawal from other people and the external world into the self that is similar to the withdrawal that Bleuler associated with autistic thinking. However, Bleuler conceived of autism not as a pathology confined to a special group of children but as a normal mode of thinking, found among children and adults alike.
> *(Harris, 2000, p. 1)*

Harris concludes in the same chapter, (which outlines the persistence of imaginative play and fantasy throughout adulthood): 'Children's ability to entertain counterfactual alternatives to an actual outcome is critical for making causal and moral judgements about that outcome' (Harris, 2000, p. 7).

And yet somehow we ended up with pathological autism in society. The implications are immense.

AUTISM AS A WAY OF BEING

Understanding autism as a way of being encourages us to celebrate the unique strengths and perspectives of autistic people and to create a more inclusive and accepting society that values neurodiversity. It reminds us that diversity in all its forms enriches our world and enhances our collective human experience. Autistic people often have a unique way of perceiving and interacting with the world. They may notice details and patterns that 'neurotypical' individuals might overlook. This different perspective can lead to innovative thinking and problem-solving. Some individuals excel in mathematics, science, music, art, or other areas, abilities which contribute significantly to various fields and industries.

As outlined above in the context of neurodiversity and social groups, the term 'predominant neurotype' (Beardon, 2017), is often used to describe the neurological traits, behaviours, and cognitive styles that are most commonly found and accepted within a particular society or culture. It is a concept that highlights the idea that there is a diversity of neurological profiles, and not all individuals fit the 'neurotypical' mould. The 'neurotypical' term is often used to refer to individuals whose neurological characteristics are in line with the majority in a given society. Autistic culture also uses the term 'allistic' as a way of describing the nature of the majority accepting that the one way of being, i.e. 'all' is a given. Autism is often contrasted with the 'neurotypical' or predominant neurotype. Autistic individuals may have different ways of thinking, processing information, and experiencing the world, which can vary significantly from what is considered typical in a particular society. Advocates of neurodiversity argue that these differences should be accepted and celebrated rather than pathologised.

So what does it mean to make *better* sense of and to each other, and how might we do that?

Many clinicians, if they are taught anything about autism, will be taught medical or deficit-based theories such as theory of mind (Baron-Cohen et al., 1985) or executive dysfunction (Damasio & Maurer, 1978; Ozonoff et al., 1991) or weak central coherence (Frith, 1989). All these theories seek to explain how autistics are different to 'normal' people because they lack something – empathy, executive functioning, the ability to see the bigger picture etc. Similarly, autism is often conflated with learning or intellectual disability (a current mainstream counselling course I saw recently referred to 'learning disabilities such as autism' epitomising this) and while the two can co-occur they are separate phenomena.

To compare here I briefly present some pioneering autism theories by autistic scientists and encourage you to look at these further – use the references provided at the end of the chapter. These theories offer an experiential and strengths-focused perspective and contribute to the aims of the Autism Dialogue Approach. Like much of the work around the evolving construct of autism, some of these theories aren't universally accepted in the mainstream field of autism research but have sparked discussion. Conversely, relatively new knowledge such as that around the specifics of autistic burnout was generated from autistic people's discussions on public internet forums and subsequently recognised by the Royal College of Psychiatrists (Johnstone & Boyle, 2018).

MONOTROPISM

Monotropism (Murray et al., 2005) describes differences in attentional style in a non-pathological way and further posits that social interactions, language and transition of attention from one thing to another are all influenced by attentional style. 'Monotropic' minds tend to give their attention deeply to a small number of interests with great depth – with the possibility of entering flow states which are intense, joyous, and often hugely productive. This is likened to an attention tunnel where there is hyper-awareness within the tunnel and hypo awareness of outside it. In contrast 'polytropic' minds will spread their attention across a wider number of interests but at less depth. Autistic/ADHD people are shown to be more likely to be monotropic (Garau et al., 2023). What is described as 'restricted patterns of interest' (American Psychiatric Association, 2013) follow from a monotropic tendency. Also, consider that it takes time to come out of a 'flow state' (Rapaport et al., 2023) which may explain why it can take an autistic person longer to transition between different activities or states. An unanticipated and unwelcome interruption for a person in an attention tunnel may be experienced as 'truly, if briefly, catastrophic:

a complete disconnection from a previous safe state, a plunge into a meaningless blizzard of sensations, a frightening experience which may occur many times in a single day' (Murray et al., 2005, p. 147). Finally, monotropism may also explain differences in communication since 'Monotropism makes it exceptionally hard to make sense of the continuous flux of social discourse' (Murray et al., 2005, p. 148). Slowing down the pace of communication in autism dialogue removes some of these barriers.

I think this theory could also easily be linked with practices which directly promote deeper states of awareness and relaxation such as mindful awareness (more on this later on).

STRESS ADAPTATION

Hogenkamp's Stress Adaptation theory (2018) suggests how stress and the need to adapt to it during critical periods of development can influence the likelihood of developing autism. Our bodies and brains are constantly adapting to stress which is to do with epigenetics. It relates to Enactivism or Enaction theory, which is rooted in biological sciences. Enactivism is a position in cognitive science that argues that cognition arises through a dynamic interaction between an acting organism and its environment, the environment of an organism is brought about, or enacted, by the active exercise of that organism's sensorimotor processes.

> Sense-making is the enactive term for cognition … our everyday making sense is intertwined with language, language is actually incorporated into all dimensions of human embodiment. We are continually in process, or becoming; we are linguistic bodies.
>
> *(Cuffari, n.d., paras 1–2)*

Hogenkamp (2018) suggests there are certain critical periods, especially during the prenatal environment and early childhood, when our brain is rapidly developing, and is more sensitive to stress and more vulnerable to environmental influences. These conditions and exposures during pregnancy, such as maternal stress, infections and exposure to certain chemicals continue with influences from early childhood environments such as poor nutrition, exposure to pollutants, and social interactions (socialisation) in the early years of life. When a person experiences stress, their brain and body try to adapt to it. If the stress is too intense or happens at a sensitive time, it might lead to changes in how the brain develops. If the brain's adaptation to stress is significant, it could contribute to the development of conditions like autism. Similarly, if anyone is exposed to environmental pollutants or nutritional deficiencies, these stressors might also lead to changes in brain development. Hogenkamp (2018) suggests that by managing stress and improving the prenatal and early childhood environment, we might reduce some of the risks associated with these environmental factors. How we do that is beyond the scope of this book but in another way, dialogic approaches suggest we can and do, especially in the examples provided by traditional societies, where autism doesn't exist.

Hogenkamp's theory suggests a unique explanation of autism and is fundamental to the explanation of how and why group Dialogue works. The theory suggests that human evolution has been shaped by our collaborative lifestyle and collective efforts within villages and communities. At the heart of early societies were the majority, composed of like-minded individuals who were predisposed to maintain harmony and cooperation. They developed the ability to manage and prioritise information in favour of social cohesion. Skilled in imitation, conformity and teamwork, they formed the core of the community. Surrounding them were less common personality types, characterised by a penchant for exploration, storytelling, and advocacy. These diverse individuals processed information differently and pursued varied goals, serving as innovators, explorers, guardians, leaders, scholars, enthusiasts, artists and creators. Despite their contrasting approaches, both the cohesive core and the diverse 'peripheral minds' contributed to our collective thriving, each bringing unique value to cooperative endeavours. This is where we begin to uncover the significance of words such as 'neurodivergent' and 'inclusion' and 'equality'.

So now we have some understanding of Hogenkamp's theory. Systemic stress upon the individual, with the onset of modernity, the industrial revolution, pollution, intensive farming, ultra-processed foods and ecosystem imbalances is when fragmentation and the *crisis of selfhood* (autism) starts. Highly sensitive people, the outliers of society are the canaries in the coal mine – the autistics. Think back to traditional societies that come together as a unit for dialogic communication and all the reasons why this might support a varied but unified system, free of stress upon any one individual.

DOUBLE EMPATHY

The double empathy problem refers to the 'mutual incomprehension that occurs between people of different dispositional outlooks and personal conceptual understandings when attempts are made to communicate meaning' (Milton, 2018). Lacking the ability to 'read between the lines' or identify subtexts of social situations is seen to be a deficit within autistic cognition. However, the double empathy theory reminds us that difficulties with communication occur across neurotypes/cultures and are due to a lack of understanding from non-autistic people to autistic people as well as the other way around. Therefore it is a double problem because both sides experience it. Yet when viewed through a deficit lens the responsibility is firmly placed on the autistic person, who is seen to have a deficit in communication. The predominant neurotype, which sees its way of interacting as 'normal' can apply a deficit label onto the 'other' whose communication is seen as incorrect. This way of thinking can lead to behavioural interventions such as social skills training designed to correct the autistic person's 'broken' style of communication. Milton (2012, p. 886) reminds us that 'it is true that autistic people often lack insight about non-AS perceptions and culture, yet it is equally the case that non-AS people lack insight into the minds and culture of autistic people. Therefore autism as a concept really is everyone's concern.

AUTISTIC COMMUNICATION STYLES

Autistic individuals often value straightforward and honest communication. They may express their thoughts and feelings with sincerity and clarity, which can be refreshing in a world where social norms sometimes obscure true intentions. Some autistic individuals may face challenges with spoken language, and yet often have rich and diverse communication styles. Nonverbal communication, such as using gestures, writing, art, or assistive technologies, can be equally expressive and meaningful. Contrary to stereotypes, many autistic individuals are highly empathetic and compassionate. They may have a deep understanding of the emotions and needs of others, even if they express it in unconventional ways. Many are hyper-empathic, which can cause further problems including overwhelm and shutdown – which to outsiders looks like the opposite and leads to assumptions of autistic people lacking empathy.

AUTISTIC PEER-TO-PEER INFORMATION TRANSFER IS HIGHLY EFFECTIVE

Crompton et al. (2020) designed a study to test one aspect of the double empathy theory. They hypothesised: 'One implication of the "double empathy problem" is that if autistic "social impairments" result from a mismatch between autistic and non-autistic populations, they may disappear in within-group interactions' (Crompton et al., 2020, p. 1705).

Results from Crompton et al.:

> autistic people recall information shared by autistic peers as effectively as non-autistic people recall information shared by non-autistic peers. Yet, information sharing is significantly poorer in chains of mixed neurotypes. These deficits in information transfer between mixed neurotype groups are accompanied by significantly poorer self-rated interactional rapport.
> *(Crompton et al., 2020, p. 1709)*

In other words, information sharing was less effective and participants felt less rapport in their communication across neurotypes than in their homogenous groups.

Non-autistic and autistic communication is seen as equal but different, and dialogue seeks to make explicit the sub consciously held 'norms' of each individual:

> In an autism dialogue, I was watching a non-autistic person across the circle who was speaking, it was like for the first time ever in real life, can you imagine, and I was amazed like they knew what to do and move and was speaking a different language, because I wasn't judging, just observing, it was almost out-of-body. I remembered a website called 'Things normals do' and laughed out loud so people looked at me.
> *(Anonymous Community ADA participant, personal communication, 2021)*

SENSORY SENSITIVITY: THE INTENSE WORLD

The Intense World Theory of Autism, proposed by neuroscientists Henry and Kamila Markram, suggests that autistic individuals experience the world with both heightened sensory perceptions and intense emotions (Markram & Markram, 2010). According to this theory, autistic individuals may have hyper-reactive brain circuits, leading to increased sensitivity and reactivity to sensory input. This can include sensitivity to sounds, textures, tastes and lights. These heightened senses can provide a deep and vivid experience of the environment. Autistic people often exhibit intense interests and passions and can immerse themselves in specific topics, hobbies or activities with remarkable dedication and expertise. Monotropism theory (Murray et al., 2005) covers this in detail (see above). Autistic individuals often find private comfort in routines and predictability, which can provide a sense of stability and security in an otherwise chaotic world.

Sensory overload is when a person's senses are overstimulated by outside stimuli. It can happen to virtually anyone. However, this sensation is most commonly seen in autistic people and those with sensory processing disorder or other neurological differences. Even though everyone has their own set of what we call symptoms (an individual's predisposed responses to a specific environment) sensory overload is common. When left unaddressed, it can significantly impact one's life. Sensory issues often go hand-in-hand with autism and can be expressed as hyper-sensitivities or hypo-sensitivities. Hypersensitivity involves heightened reactions to one's sensory environment (i.e., the need to cover their ears when someone sings or when hearing an emergency siren).

Hyposensitivity involves behaviours that are lowered reactions to one's environment (i.e., not responding to a loud sound). These sensitivities will be associated with a wide array of stimuli, ranging from sights and sounds to smells and tastes. For example, many autistic people experience hypersensitivity to bright lights. Other people may find the sensation of touch incredibly uncomfortable. Sensory sensitivity can also be affected by other factors such as tiredness, stress and mood fluctuations. So the sensory experience is completely unique to each individual but also varies for each individual.

Sensory overload is usually directed to your five senses but can also be social and relational. There are many subtler effects of being with other people, and countless ways both they and the environment communicate to us, with us and also from us, in a never-ending feedback loop. At times of sensory overload, the brain is overwhelmed by all this input – taking in more information at a time than your brain can process. We can then enter into fight, flight or freeze mode in response to what feels like a crisis, which makes us feel unsafe and overwhelmed.

In contrast, sensory seeking often occurs when there's a need for calibration.

MASKING

'Masking' was recognised by the Greeks and Romans and in Renaissance Italy in poetry and theatre, as aligning with the instinct of imitation, then later to hide one's true identity (to escape being recognised and punished for breaking the law or having a good time). Twentieth-century psychology literature recognised it as something we all do as an escape or a coping mechanism – like not swearing in front of our parents. However, autistic masking has to do with psychological survival and is generally more impactful, especially in the long term (Radulski, 2022).

In a group dialogue context, autistic masking can deeply impact both the individual masking and the overall group dynamics. When someone masks, they suppress their natural communication style and behaviours to fit in with neurotypical norms, often for self-protection or to avoid judgement or discomfort, rather than by choice. This process is mentally exhausting, leading to emotional fatigue and a limited ability to engage fully. Over time, the individual may struggle to contribute authentically, which reduces their presence in the dialogue and diminishes the richness of the conversation.

Masking also affects self-expression. The person may filter their thoughts, feelings and responses to align with what they think others expect, which can prevent their true voice from being heard. This can cause them to feel disconnected from the group and others may sense that something is being withheld, subtly affecting trust and cohesion. The group might miss out on the unique insights and perspectives that could emerge if the individual felt free to express themselves fully. The constant monitoring and modification of behaviour can heighten anxiety, making it difficult for the person masking to be fully present or to explore more vulnerable or personal aspects of the conversation. This affects the depth of the dialogue and can prevent the emergence of new insights or creative solutions.

From the group's perspective, if they are unaware of the masking, they might unconsciously perpetuate social norms that favour certain communication styles, making the space feel less inclusive. This can stifle the generative potential of the group, as diverse forms of expression are key to transformative dialogue. To create a more inclusive and supportive environment, facilitators should foster an atmosphere where diverse communication styles are not just accepted but valued. This could include allowing for silence, encouraging authenticity, stimming, and being mindful of different pacing and forms of interaction.

Addressing the implications of autistic masking in group dialogue requires creating a safe space where everyone feels comfortable being themselves. This not only supports the individual masking but also enhances the overall generative potential of the dialogue, allowing for a richer, more inclusive exchange of ideas.

TRAUMA – AN INTRODUCTION

Autistic people may be criticised or punished for acting in ways which don't conform to social expectations. For example, autistic people often do not understand, see or accept typical hierarchies and may treat a teacher or police officer in the same way as they would a sibling, friend or peer. Seeing this as rude, arrogant or threatening is a misinterpretation of their intentions and behaviours and frequently results in negative reactions which can impact their mental health.

Autistic people can face many other unique challenges and stressors that may have negative effects on their mental health. They may struggle with social interactions, leading to othering, isolation and loneliness, making it harder for them to form and maintain relationships. They are at an increased risk of being bullied or stigmatised due to their differences. They may have heightened sensory sensitivities, which can lead to anxiety and stress in environments with excessive sensory stimuli. Sensory overload can be overwhelming and lead to meltdowns or shutdowns. For non-speaking autistic people, communicating their needs and feelings can be challenging when alternative forms of communication are not enabled. This frustration can lead to feelings of helplessness and agitation. Communication difficulties and differences can lead to othering, exclusion, loneliness, feelings of sadness, depression, and anxiety and these are major contributors to self-harm, suicidal ideation and suicide (Cassidy et al., 2022).

OTHER PROBLEMS THAT AUTISTIC INDIVIDUALS MAY FACE

- Rejection or misunderstanding from peers, teachers, employers, or healthcare providers who are not knowledgeable about their specific needs and strengths
- Co-occurring mental health conditions such as depression, anxiety disorders, and attention deficit disorders and reduced access to mental health services or therapies tailored to their needs due to lack of awareness or resources
- Internalised societal stereotypes or negative attitudes about their condition, leading to self-stigma, internalised ableism and reduced self-esteem
- Major life transitions, such as moving from school to work or living independently, can be particularly challenging, leading to increased stress and uncertainty

It is important to note that while autistic individuals may face these challenges, like all humans, they also possess unique strengths and abilities. Advocates of autistics emphasise the importance of recognising and building upon unique strengths to support the wellbeing of autistic individuals. Providing a supportive and inclusive environment, raising awareness, and offering tailored interventions and accommodations can all contribute to better mental health outcomes for autistics.

Viewing autism as a way of being reminds us that being neurologically different is not a deficit but rather a distinct way of experiencing and contributing to the world. Autistic individuals have much to offer in terms of their perspectives, talents, and insights.

THE NEED FOR DIALOGUES IN AUTISM

I suggest there is a strong connection between some autistic-led social scientific theories, environmental factors (which we are implicit in) and oppression by our ruling classes (explicit).

The connection between these theories and the concept of oppression by the ruling class is perhaps more abstract or philosophically in-depth than we can cover in this book. However, some advocates of autistic identity argue that societal norms and expectations, which are often defined and enforced by those in positions of power (the ruling class), can marginalise and oppress autistic people. The emphasis on conformity to a 'predominant neurotype' can perpetuate discrimination and inequality, and we know there is bullying and ostracising of autistic children from their early playground experiences.

REFERENCES

American Psychiatric Association. (2013). *Diagnostic and Statistical Manual of Mental Disorders* (5th ed.). https://doi.org/10.1176/appi.books.9780890425596

Baron-Cohen, S., Leslie, A. M. & Frith, U. (1985). Does the autistic child have a 'theory of mind'? Cognition, 21(1), 37–46. https://doi.org/10.1016/0010-0277(85)90022-8

Beardon, L. (2017). *Autism and Asperger Syndrome in Adults*. Sheldon Press.

Bleuler, E. (1950 [1911]). *Dementia Praecox or the Group of Schizophrenias*. International Universities.

Cassidy, S., et al. (2022). Autism and autistic traits in those who died by suicide in England. The British Journal of Psychiatry, 221(5), 683–691. https://doi.org/10.1192/bjp.2022.21

Crompton, C. J., Ropar, D., Evans-Williams, C. V., Flynn, E. G. & Fletcher-Watson, S. (2020). Autistic peer-to-peer information transfer is highly effective. Autism. https://doi.org/10.1177/1362361320919286

Cuffari, E. E. (n.d.). What does it mean to make sense? Retrieved from www.elenaclarecuffari.com/research

Damasio, A. R. & Maurer, R. G. (1978). Neurological model for childhood autism. Archives of Neurology, 35, 777–1286.

Frith, U. (1989). *Autism: Explaining the Enigma*. Blackwell.

Garau, V., Murray, A., Woods, R., Chown, N., Hallett, S., Murray, F., Wood, R. & Fletcher-Watson, S. (2023). Development and validation of a novel self-report measure of monotropism in autistic and non-autistic people: the monotropism questionnaire. Retrieved from https://osf.io/preprints/osf/ft73y

Harris, L. P. (2000). *The Work of the Imagination (Understanding Children's Worlds)*. Wiley-Blackwell.

Hogenkamp, L. (2018). Is autism a stress adaptation of neurodivergent neurotypes? Peripheral minds of autism. https://peripheralmindsofautism.com/2018/04/17/is-autism-a-stress-adaptation/

Holt, A. (2019). The conversation: feedback structures, ways of knowing, and neurodivergence. Public, 30(59), 104–112. https://doi.org/10.1386/public.30.59.104_1

Johnstone, L. & Boyle, M. (2018). *The Power Threat Meaning Framework: Towards the Identification of Patterns in Emotional Distress, Unusual Experiences and Troubled or Troubling Behaviour, as an Alternative to Functional Psychiatric Diagnosis*. British Psychological Society.

Kanner, L. (1943). Autistic disturbances of affective contact. Nervous Child, 2, 217–250.

Markram, K. & Markram, H. (2010). The intense world theory – a unifying theory of the neurobiology of autism. Frontiers in Human Neuroscience 4: 224 https://doi.org/10.3389/fnhum.2010.00224

Milton, D. (2012). On the ontological status of autism: the 'double empathy problem'. Disability and Society, 27(3), 883–887.

Milton, D. E. M. (2018). From finding voice to being understood: exploring the double empathy problem. Retrieved from www.autscape.org/2013/programme/handouts/Double%20empathy%20problem.pdf

Murray, D., Lesser, M. & Lawson, W. (2005). Attention, monotropism and the diagnostic criteria for autism. Autism, 9(2), 139–156. https://doi.org/10.1177/1362361305051398

Ozonoff, S., Pennington, B. F. & Rogers, S. J. (1991). Executive function deficits in high-functioning autistic individuals: relationship to theory of mind. Journal of Child Psychology, Psychiatry and Allied Disciplines, 32, 1081–1105.

Radulski, E. M. (2022). Conceptualising autistic masking, camouflaging, and neurotypical privilege: towards a minority group model of neurodiversity. Human Development, 66(2), 113–127. https://doi.org/10.1159/000524122

Rapaport, H., Clapham, H., Adams, J., Lawson, W., Porayska-Pomsta, K. & Pellicano, E. (2024). 'In a state of flow': a qualitative examination of autistic adults' phenomenological experiences of task immersion. Autism in Adulthood, 6(3), 362–373. https://doi.org/10.1089/aut.2023.0032

CHAPTER 7

Autism and Dialogue through the lens of social sciences

Much of our thinking happens unconsciously, beyond our direct, conscious awareness. The mental processes that shape our thoughts and language occur so quickly and at such a deep level that they are difficult to observe directly. Abstract ideas are often rooted in metaphor, and many key philosophical concepts such as time, morality, causation, the mind and the self – are shaped by fundamental metaphors grounded in our bodily experiences. Take hypersensitivity, a very common trait in autistic people, which refers to a (relatively) unfiltered experience, whatever that experience is (Manning, 2018). But it's possible when you hear the word 'hypersensitive' you sense something negative. Why is this, when the person is literally part of, and so responding to their environment?

We all exist in relation to each other, so one person can't be simply autistic, somehow as an individual isolated fragment, disassociated from everything and everyone else. As a creative, I often wonder what radical approaches, thinking, acts and processes can dislodge society's negative feedback loops, disrupt ideologies which conflict and negate, and what implications there are for other minority groups stuck in unfair power structures.

According to the social model, disability is dynamic, the environment is as much a disabling factor and in autism, an individual's sense of self (autos) is determined equally by both their inner and outer environments, self and other, and the relationship between them. Conflict in societal definitions persists and autism's meaning has largely developed under technocratic power structures; 'within capitalism, the Autism Industrial Complex (AIC) produces both autism as commodity and the normative cultural logic of intervention in relation to it' (Broderick & Roscigno, 2021, p. 77).

Autism manifests as inequalities, social struggles, much higher rates of unemployment, poor mental health, loneliness and suicide, than in the non-autistic population (Autistica, n.d.) and autistic researcher Nick Chown tells us:

> It is both epistemologically, as well as ethically, problematic if the autistic voice is not heard in relation to social scientific research seeking to further develop knowledge of autism. Ever since autism first emerged, it has remained medicalised and almost exclusively the preserve of non-autistic researchers.
>
> *(Chown et al., 2017)*

Dominating value systems and deficit narratives persist, permeating language and maintaining power-over, so that communication and meaning-making is not equally participatory and the minority side must be permanently disadvantaged. Society's ableism and normalcy, argues Professor Nick Hodge, are 'the twin evils that decide some bodies have more value than others and that your body has to look and behave a certain way to be deemed acceptable, still control the cultural norms' (Hodge, 2017, p. 15). Autistic researcher Damian Milton describes the 'double empathy problem' as a breach in the 'natural attitude' that occurs between people of different dispositional outlooks and personal conceptual understandings when attempts are made to communicate meaning – based in the social interaction between two differently disposed social actors' (Milton, 2012, p. 884) and crucially, emphasis is on majority conformity and assumptions of unspoken social rules.

Autism researcher Professor Matthew Belmonte suggests it's the categorical nature of language which falsifies the more complex and shaded reality of the autism spectrum, contributing to domination of spaces, conflict, social inequity, exclusion, othering, isolation, loneliness and complex trauma (Belmonte, 2017). We know that the effects of all this in turn contribute to a lifetime of masking, self-harm and suicide (Autistica, n.d.).

The term *atopos*, meaning 'strange' or 'out of place,' closely parallels autism in its etymological roots, as both words evoke a sense of spatial dislocation. *Atopos* is also the root of words like *atopia*, which conveys the idea of a world without borders (Foucault, 1995), and *autopoiesis* (see section below) from the words self and creation. The spatial metaphor can serve as a lens through which to examine the discourse of autism in cultural narratives, particularly those featuring personal accounts of autistic individuals. The word autism suggests existence is restricted to the self but to be autistic is not to be self-enclosed, but open and potentially vulnerable to all sorts of outside influences (McGrath, 2017). In online spaces particularly, abstractions of relationships and notions of friendship persist, so both are dissolved. We are negatively affected by computational algorithms in popular media too, which is dominated by deficit narratives and technocratic ideologies. In these narratives, creative negotiations and crossings of space – whether physical, social, or discursive – are central themes (Deleuze & Guattari, 1987). This counter-metaphor introduces a new perspective on autistic bodies and identities, proposing that they are continuously shaped by the interplay between bodies and the discursive spaces they inhabit.

In my own personal and professional life, as well as avoiding popular television and radio, I've learned to develop my intuition and, concerning people, this means to help them rather than (or as well as) protect myself from them. From *interbeing* (Buddhism, etc.) to enactivism and participatory sense-making (social cognitive science) we are linguistic bodies (Di Paolo et al., 2018) – constantly interacting, reacting and responding to and with everything.

Dr Hanne De Jaegher has developed participatory sense-making, which happens when we participate in each other's precarious processes of sense-making 'but also of the interaction process, which is also autonomous and thus precarious ... This makes it possible to deeply affect one another and requires us to navigate tensions between embodied and interactive normative domains that are not guaranteed to be in alignment' (De Jaegher, 2019, p. 855).

So as we're all constantly enacting and interacting, we may ask, what is knowing?

> But thought thinks it's a problem out there and I must solve it. That doesn't make sense because simultaneously thought is doing all the things which make the problem and then tries to do another set of activities to try and overcome it.
> *(Bohm, 1990, cited by Chase, 2014, para. 7)*

Dialogue is an opportunity to explore these questions. Language can be more interesting and potent when used as a dynamic and culturally sensitive meaning-making process (Manning, 2010).

NATURE OF SELF

The classical Western cultural definition of the self is rooted in the traditions of ancient Greek philosophy, particularly in the works of thinkers like Plato, and Aristotle, and later in the writings of figures like Descartes during the so-called Enlightenment. The classical view emphasises the self as a rational, individual entity characterised by consciousness, identity and personal agency, and has shaped the understanding of personhood, identity and morality in Western societies. Western thought places a strong emphasis on individual identity, wherein the self is viewed as a distinct, autonomous individual with personal rights, moral agency, and responsibility for actions. The concept of free will is closely tied to this view, suggesting that everyone can make choices that are truly their own. Particularly in the tradition of Aristotle, the self in the West is primarily defined by reason, central to this concept is our ability to think rationally, make decisions, and seek knowledge. Further to this, when Descartes famously declared 'Cogito, ergo sum' ('I think, therefore I am') in 1637, emphasising that the self is fundamentally a thinking, conscious entity distinct from the body, he separated the self into mind (thinking-self) and body (physical matter of self), and established dualism and the fragmentation of consciousness. This paradigm reigns over most of society to this day.

Dominated by concepts of freedom, modernity and emphasis on the individual, Western society emphasises personal autonomy, self-expression and the pursuit of individual goals, viewing the self as an independent entity with unique rights and responsibilities. In contrast, Eastern cultures, particularly in traditions influenced by Confucianism, Buddhism, Sufism and other communal wisdom traditions and philosophies, prioritise the wellbeing and harmony of the group. Here, the self is seen as interconnected, with identity closely tied to relationships, family, and societal roles. While Western individualism values personal freedom and self-determination, Eastern traditions emphasise collective duty, social cohesion and the importance of contributing to the greater whole.

Whether Western individual or Eastern communal, the growth to attaining selfhood is a universal concept, and transforming our ordinary self and transcending its limitations requires deliberate and dedicated effort. In this process, Eastern cultures espouse that sincere religious or spiritual belief and practice can serve as a transitional pathway for personal growth, with practice, method and religion, therefore, becoming a starting point. Depending on the spiritual state of the *self-seeker*, traditional religious belief can foster identification with the Self/Creator/Tao etc. or at least with its attributes. That is a journey which brings the seeker to the edge of self-realisation, to a moment of resolution and commitment. At this point, intellectual knowledge, conceptualisation, and Aristotelian logic prove inadequate. Many wisdom traditions have developed a dual approach, combining behavioural discipline and inner experience under the guidance of a teacher, to achieve selfhood and affirm it through a deeper experience of what has been called the climax of being, 'where knowledge and conceptualization and Aristotelian logic are found to be helpless' (Reza Arasteh, 1988, p xii).

DIALOGUE AS A SYSTEM

Other theories can be helpful in understanding how Dialogue works and how it is relevant to the outside world. Systems theory views the universe as an interconnected whole, or as a complex system of interacting parts; it emphasises that properties and behaviours emerge from these interactions that cannot be predicted by examining individual components alone. Complexity theory deals with how simple interactions can lead to complex behaviours and patterns and is often used to understand natural phenomena like weather systems, ecosystems, and even the behaviour of social groups. Thought is a system and Bohm explains that dispute, division and violence exist because of a deep and pervasive defect in the process of human thought (Bohm et al., 1991).

Biologists Francisco Varela, Humberto Maturana and Rodrigo Uribe developed the idea of Autopoietic systems as a unity that undergoes dynamic, self-referential interactions (such as metabolism) while creating a boundary (such as the cell membrane) (Varela et al., 1987, p. 46).

Autopoiesis is at the core of an enactive understanding of life, as it specifies the kind of organisational pattern exhibited by all living beings. In this context, the self-organising universe (system) is seen as inherently creative and resilient. Order and harmony can emerge naturally from within the system rather than being imposed externally. This is crucial in considering the position and attitude of dialogue *facilitation*, which means making something easier. This idea contrasts with traditional views of a mechanistic universe where external forces drive change, as in the monologue of an information provider or tutor/teacher. The self-organising universe presents a dynamic, interconnected web of relationships where each part influences, and is influenced by the whole. These relationship webs are also known as regenerating systems or self-organising systems, and that's what a group dialogue essentially is, or aims towards becoming, aided by the process of all participants aiming to facilitate that process.

The theory of participatory sense-making (Cuffari et al., 2015) builds upon the enactive approach and social sciences which includes systems thinking. In *The Embodied Mind*, Varela, Thompson and Rosch (1991) provide a unique, sophisticated view of the spontaneous and reflective dimension of human experience. Participatory sense-making, rooted in Enactive theory, examines social interaction processes in subjectivity and intersubjectivity, examining the connections between how we interact and communicate together, how we influence and understand each other and the world (together) and how all that makes us who we are. Enactivism suggests that only by having a sense of common ground between both mind in science and mind in experience can our understanding of cognition be a more complete and more harmonious system of human knowledge and understanding. In a similar vein, Bohm presents this as a possibility:

> We are internally related to everything, not externally related. Consciousness is an internal relationship to the whole, we take in the whole, and we act toward the whole. Whatever we have taken in determines basically what we are. Wholeness is a kind of attitude or approach to the whole of life. If we can have a coherent approach to reality then reality will respond coherently to us.
> *(Bohm, 1990, cited by Chase, 2014, para 3)*

Varela's theory instigated many significant dialogues between cognitive social scientists and Buddhists. With the Dalai Lama, Varela co-founded the Mind and Life organisation, which is increasingly active in the domain of contemplative science, situating Enactivism and Buddhism in relation to other western traditions such as phenomenology and psychotherapy.

LETTING BE, THINKING, PARTICIPATORY SENSE-MAKING AND GENERATIVE DIALOGUE

In De Jaegher's paper 'Loving and Knowing: Reflections for an Engaged Epistemology' (2019) we find a suitable ontological description for generative dialogue, which is seen as the highest form of Dialogue. Working at the intersection of psychology, philosophy, neuroscience, linguistics and computer science, Dr De Jaegher provides an interdisciplinary scientific basis for beliefs and praxis that life is all to do with learning together. De Jaegher (2019) posits that we are each the result of a long and continuous process of collaborative learning, and any relationship worth having is a learning process, which changes us and our environment.

Cognitive social science moves us away from the so-called Theory of Mind (one of the refuted 'triad of impairments' in autism) which in short, states that our brain works like a computer (and that autistic people are lacking in this area). The 'input, transformation, output' basis for this theory was proposed by Descartes in the 17th century, who made a radical distinction between our brains and the world around us. This view continues to influence the mindset of the 'predominant neurotype' in our modern, western society, whose values and sense of meaning are aligned with the nomothetic (general) rather than the idiographic (unique) (Milton, 2012). This dominant frame of reference, and the fact that autism originates from the 'non-autistic' perspective, is ontologically problematic; yet science holds a widely prevalent superstition that interest in the so-called fringe areas of dialogue, the transpersonal and relational is 'a sign of woolly thinking and declining intellectual vigour' (Ramachandran, 1980).

De Jaegher (2019) argues that understanding knowledge, especially in a social context, requires recognising the essential role of interactions. According to enactivism, cognition isn't just an internal process but something that unfolds in the interactions between people and their environment. In this framework, knowing is deeply relational and emerges from the dynamic, reciprocal engagement with others. We can do many things on our own but it is pairs of people learning about each other who fall in love and groups of people learning together who form communities. As mentioned, many communities are based on the premise of loving and knowing being inseparable. Participatory sense-making happens when agents participate in each other's sense-making, allowing for significant mutual influence, as in human loving, and requires us to manage tensions between embodied and interactive norms that may not necessarily align (Cuffari et al., 2015).

BOHM'S THEORY OF WHOLENESS AND THE IMPLICATE ORDER

Bohm's theory of Wholeness and the Implicate Order (1980) is a groundbreaking framework that provides an alternative perspective on the nature of reality and the interconnectedness of the universe, which continues to influence physics, philosophy, metaphysics, social science, and increasingly, organisational development and human communication. Bohm proposed that there is an underlying unity that transcends the apparent diversity and fragmentation we perceive in the world and at the most fundamental level of reality, the universe is in a state of constant and dynamic motion, which Bohm termed the 'holomovement'. The holomovement suggests that all things, from subatomic particles to galaxies, are in a perpetual state of flux, vibrating and interacting with one another. Also central to Bohm's philosophy is the concept of the 'Implicate Order', the hidden, enfolded structure of reality that underlies the apparent diversity and fragmentation of the world. In the Implicate Order, everything is interconnected and interrelated. The entire universe is one indivisible whole, with each part containing information about the whole.

In contrast to the Implicate Order, Bohm (1980) also introduced the idea of the 'Explicate Order', which is the observable, manifest world that we perceive through our senses. The Explicate Order is a projection of the deeper, hidden reality of the Implicate Order. It represents the unfolded, apparent world of separate entities. Bohm emphasised the interplay between order and disorder in the universe, suggesting order arises from the implicit, interconnected structure of the Implicate Order, while disorder emerges in the explicit, separate manifestations of the Explicate Order. According to Bohm, many of the challenges and problems in the world result from a lack of understanding of the inherent unity in the Implicate Order. Bohm's holistic view of the universe stands in opposition to the mechanistic science of Newton and Aristotle and as far from Cartesian reductionism as any science could be.

Artist Hester Reeve, whose research encompasses live art, philosophy, drawing and social sculpture, introduced Bohm Dialogue as a research model into the Contemporary Fine Art degree when I was studying at Sheffield Hallam University's Institute of Arts and Design. Over the many years since its inception as the Sheffield School of Art in 1837, the organisation has opened up a much broader definition of the artist, presenting it in terms of the relationship between human agency and critical thinking – an ethos which aligns with my sense of the need for engaging creative approaches (art) directly into society.

Dialogue is socially creative because it involves the co-construction of meaning and the generation of new ideas through interaction. Participants bring their unique perspectives, experiences and insights, which combine in ways that lead to new understandings or solutions that no single individual could achieve alone. The process is inherently creative because it relies on active listening, adapting to others' viewpoints and collaboratively exploring possibilities. Dialogue fosters relationships and shared knowledge, making it a powerful tool for building community, innovation and collective growth. In the context of social justice, dialogue is crucial for addressing power imbalances and amplifying marginalised voices. It enables communities to collectively recognise and dismantle systemic injustices, while also building inclusive frameworks for equity and change. By prioritising listening, empathy, and shared humanity, dialogue becomes a transformative tool for achieving social justice goals.

Because it is based on a design that emphasises equity, dialogue creates solutions which are inclusive, participatory and socially just. It emphasises the co-creation of ideas and solutions through deep, respectful conversations among diverse stakeholders, particularly those who are traditionally marginalised or underrepresented. The goal is to ensure that all voices are heard and valued equally in the design process, fostering outcomes that reflect the needs and experiences of everyone involved, especially those who are most impacted. Socially engaged dialogue also involves power awareness; recognising and addressing power imbalances to prevent any single group (or individual) from dominating.

SYSTEMIC TRAUMA

Systemic trauma refers to the widespread and ongoing harm caused by structural inequalities, discriminatory practices, and societal systems that perpetuate marginalisation and oppression. It is embedded within institutions, cultural norms, and social policies that continuously disadvantage certain groups, leading to long-term psychological, emotional, and social consequences. It affects everyone.

For autistic people, systemic trauma often manifests through repeated experiences of exclusion, misunderstanding and mistreatment within environments that are not designed to accommodate their needs (Pearson et al., 2023). This includes barriers in education, healthcare, employment, and social interactions, where societal norms and expectations are misaligned with neurodivergent ways of thinking and behaving. Autistic individuals may face stigma, ableism, and a lack of support, resulting in chronic stress, anxiety, and a sense of alienation.

The cumulative impacts of a result of systemic trauma can lead to a deep sense of disempowerment and mistrust, making it harder for autistic people to fully participate in society and access necessary resources.

Dialogue creates spaces for people to come together, share experiences and offer peer support, allowing participants to connect with others who have faced similar traumas. The shared space helps reduce feelings of isolation, shame, and self-blame. Individuals receive validation of their feelings and experiences, which is crucial for those who may have been dismissed or invalidated in the past. Tailored group Dialogue can address cultural sensitivities and is crucial for intersectional mental health and autistic trauma. Dialogue's open exchange fosters a safe environment for expressing and processing emotions. Tools like mindfulness, relaxation techniques, and improved communication skills empower individuals to take control of their healing, gaining confidence in managing trauma. As Dialogue becomes more widespread, mental health support is increasingly accessible, reducing stigma and fostering community networks that advocate for trauma awareness and societal change.

Dialogue promotes collective growth, impacting not just personal healing but broader social structures, possibly aiding trauma and healing on individual, systemic, and societal levels. Viewing nature as a self-organising system and oneself as intrinsic to it, emphasises the importance of unity in all diversity. Dialogue creates the container for genuinely inclusive environments that support wellbeing for all, regardless of type.

In embracing the self-organising principle (Ashby, 1947) together with the praxis of Bohm Dialogue and participatory sense-making, we find profound insights and practical tools for fostering harmony and understanding, particularly among negatively impacted autistic individuals. Dialogue, in the way I mean it, is a radical and practical activity, which aims to disturb and reorient, and relieve autistic suffering, rather than give in to normative logic. In Dialogue, we work without an agenda at the very edges of meaning, as close to the edge as we can (safely) get. If there is to be an agenda it is of care and generosity. The challenge then, comes when we return to the 'outside world' and want or need to quantify and qualify Dialogue, especially by using existing social and scientific frameworks and modernist mindsets such as evaluation. The word 'evaluation' itself is from the Greek meaning *value/strong,* which implicitly, therefore, seeks to maintain the status quo and existing definitions and structures of power and dominance, through thought and language. These deeply set patterns play out in dialogue through our beliefs, assumptions and language, and thus provide the tensions with which we must work, perhaps asking 'what are we thinking together?'

Sociological theories have yet to significantly influence values-led activities but applying phenomenological concepts, for example, can reveal the limitless potential for creativity by challenging and transcending our assumed social structures and constraints. Phenomenology posits that individuals possess a shared knowledge base that forms their reality, a reality taken for granted and learned through social interaction. Shared knowledge creates the assumption that everyone experiences the same world; however, what we perceive as real is not inherently so.

We live on the blurred lines between the individual and social and as such, we are constantly enacting a sort of collective unconscious and the idea Descartes and Newton presented us with, of a world that can be reduced to pieces, is dead. In terms of social cognitive science like enactivism and participatory sense-making, knowledge and knowing is embraced as an ecology of life. Dialogue as praxis enables a slow 'peeling back' of our conditioning by fragmented and polarising tendencies (and to deny that one person's views are fully isolated is the greatest fallacy). This is why in Dialogue we all need to be careful not to isolate each other with reductionist forms of knowing and intelligence – that's part of its purpose. As a person labelled by a normative society as autistic, I don't buy it, nor its tendencies for being quick to reduce, name, compartmentalise and categorise. Our stuck and traumatised systems wear *meta-masks*, and tend to prefer semantical division over dynamic meaning-making. Fights for social justice require radical new ways of understanding – together.

LOCKDOWN

Let's take a look at how autistic people were impacted by a major social event in our time, the pandemic lockdown. For many autistic people, the COVID-19 pandemic presented magnified challenges and experiences related to human connection. While some may have found relief in the reduced social demands brought about by lockdowns (no longer in a minority as a 'recluse') and social distancing (no more unwanted hugs), others may have struggled with the abrupt disruption of routines and the loss of familiar social structures. For the many autistic people who rely heavily on routine and predictability, the sudden changes brought about by the pandemic were particularly distressing – mental health dramatically declined and self-harm and suicide rates went up (National Autistic Society, 2020). The shift to remote communication and virtual interactions may have posed difficulties for some autistic individuals who thrive on face-to-face communication or who struggle with nonverbal cues often lost in digital interactions. The loss of in-person social opportunities was acutely felt by many autistic individuals who value these connections but already face barriers to forming and maintaining them, due to social challenges associated with autism (National Autistic Society, 2020). However, amidst these challenges, there may have also been moments of resilience and adaptation. Some autistics may have found comfort in the increased flexibility of remote communication, while others may have discovered new ways to connect with peers online or to engage in activities of interest from the safety of their homes.

As society has emerged from the pandemic, there is an opportunity to reflect on how to better support the diverse needs of autistic people in times of crisis and beyond. This may involve considering the ways in which virtual communication and social interactions can be made more accessible and inclusive, as well as recognising the importance of providing support and resources to help autistics navigate changes and disruptions to their routines and social environments.

Fostering human connection might involve finding ways to accommodate sensory sensitivities during gatherings, such as providing quiet spaces or allowing for breaks when needed. It could also mean embracing alternative forms of communication, such as written messages or structured activities, to facilitate interaction and engagement. Creating a supportive and understanding environment where autistics feel accepted and valued for who they are can significantly enhance their sense of belonging and connection. This may involve promoting neurodiversity awareness and providing resources and accommodations to help autistic people participate more fully in social activities. Ultimately, by recognising and respecting the unique needs and preferences of autistic individuals, we can create more inclusive and meaningful opportunities for connection and community, enriching the lives of all involved. 'The properties of mind are not purely mental: They are shaped in crucial ways by the body and brain and how the body can function in everyday life. The embodied mind is thus very much of this world' (Lakoff & Johnson, 1999, p. 565).

Enaction theory impacts on the role of consciousness, highlighting the importance of embodied communication and awareness, and whilst it may seem strange to point out the obvious, mindful awareness is central to relating and communicating. The role of consciousness in communication breakdown relates to the idea that our subjective experiences and awareness influence how we interpret and respond to messages. In the digital world, people often multitask, leading to divided attention and reduced awareness of the nuances in communication. This can result in misunderstandings and misinterpretations.

HOW CAN DIALOGUE ADDRESS COMMUNICATION BREAKDOWN?

In the digital age, algorithms, echo chambers and filter bubbles cause internet users to encounter only information and opinions that conform to and reinforce their own beliefs, that personalise the online experience. This can limit exposure to diverse perspectives, hindering meaningful dialogue and fostering social fragmentation. By contrast, Dialogism theory emphasises the dynamic, interactive nature of language and the need for diverse dialogues (Bakhtin, 1981).

Meaning is co-constructed through dialogue between individuals (Coghlan & Brydon-Miller, 2014). As covered earlier in this chapter, Bohm's (1980) theory of wholeness and the implicate order posits that everything is interconnected at a fundamental level and underscores the interconnectedness of society. Applied to social fragmentation, the theory suggests that when communication becomes fragmented and divisive, it disrupts the larger societal order and harmony and can lead to polarisation and social isolation. So does fragmentation of communication lie within the default way we view the world?

> [I]t is argued by Positivists that there exists regularities in the social world that can be observed and measured; that researchers can distinguish between value judgements and factual statements; and so in epistemological terms, knowledge is seen to be empirically testable.
>
> *(Milton & Moon, 2012)*

The foundation of the scientific method is the idea that nature operates independently of human perspectives or purposes. Scientists believe that you can't truly understand the world by assuming things happen for a specific purpose or final goal. Instead, science focuses on observable facts and evidence, not on speculating about deeper meanings or purposes that can't be proven. Many scientists avoid exploring topics beyond what can be measured or demonstrated and this infects everything. Modern communication breakdown and social fragmentation are multifaceted issues influenced by the digital age's transformative effects on language and interaction. Addressing these challenges requires a holistic approach that recognises the interplay of these factors.

REFERENCES

Ashby, W. R. (1947). Principles of the self-organizing dynamic system. The Journal of General Psychology, 37(2), 125–128. https://doi.org/10.1080/00221309.1947.9918144

Autistica. (n.d.). Suicide and autism. Retrieved from www.autistica.org.uk/what-is-autism/suicide-and-autism

Bakhtin, M. (1981). *The Dialogic Imagination*. University of Texas Press.

Belmonte, M. (2017). The categorical nature of language falsifies autism. Retrieved from https://autismdialogue.wordpress.com/testimonial/257/

Bohm, D. (1980). *Wholeness and the Implicate Order*. Routledge & Kegan Paul.

Bohm, D., Factor, D. & Garrett, P. (1991). Dialogue – a proposal. Retrieved from https://aofpd.org/library/public-resources/dialogue-a-proposal

Broderick, A. & Roscigno, R. (2021). Autism, Inc.: the autism industrial complex. Journal of Disability Studies in Education. 2. 1–25. 10.1163/25888803-bja10008. https://brill.com/view/journals/jdse/2/1/article-p77_77.xml

Chase, C. (2014). Wholeness: a coherent approach to reality – David Bohm. Retrieved from https://creativesystemsthinking.wordpress.com/2014/10/01/wholeness-a-coherent-approach-to-reality-david-bohm/

Chown, N., et al. (2017). Improving research about us, with us: a draft framework for inclusive autism research. Disability & Society, 32(5), 720–734. https://doi.org/10.1080/09687599.2017.1320273

Coghlan, D., & Brydon-Miller, M. (2014). Bakhtinian dialogism. In *The Sage Encyclopedia of Action Research* (vol. 2, pp. 73–75). Sage. https://doi.org/10.4135/9781446294406

Cuffari, E. C., Di Paolo, E. & De Jaegher, H. (2015). From participatory sense-making to language: there and back again. Phenomenology and the Cognitive Sciences, 14, 1089–1125. https://doi.org/10.1007/s11097-014-9404-9

De Jaegher, H. (2019). Loving and knowing: reflections for an engaged epistemology. Phenomenology and the Cognitive Sciences, 20(5), 847–870. https://doi.org/10.1007/s11097-019-09634-5

Deleuze, G. & Guattari, F. (1987). *A Thousand Plateaus: Capitalism and Schizophrenia.* University of Minnesota Press.

Descartes, R. (1986). *Discourse on Method.* Macmillan.

Di Paolo, E., De Jaegher, H. & Cuffari, E. (2018). *Linguistic Bodies: The Continuity between Life and Language.* MIT Press.

Foucault, M. (1995). *Discipline and Punish: The Birth of the Prison.* Vintage Books.

Hodge, N. (2017). Developing the rights approach for autism. Professorial inaugural lecture Retrieved from https://theautismcentre.files.wordpress.com/2017/03/rights-approach-for-autism-hodge.doc

Lakoff, G. & Johnson, M. (1999) *Philosophy in the Flesh: The Embodied Mind and its Challenges to Western Thought.* University of Chicago Press.

McGrath, J. (2017). *Naming Adult Autism: Culture, Science, Identity.* Rowman & Littlefield.

Manning, E. (2010). Always more than one: the collectivity of a *life.* Body & Society, 16(1). https://doi.org/10.1177/1357034X09354128

Manning, E. (2018). Histories of violence: neurodiversity and the policing of the norm. Retrieved from https://lareviewofbooks.org/article/histories-of-violence-neurodiversity-and-the-policing-of-the-norm

Milton, D. (2012). On the Ontological Status of Autism: the 'Double Empathy Problem. Disability and Society, 27(3), 883–887.

Milton, D. & Moon, L. (2012). The normalisation agenda and the psycho-emotional disablement of autistic people. Retrieved from www.larry-arnold.net/Autonomy/article/AR3/

National Autistic Society. (2020). Left stranded: the impact of coronavirus on autistic people and families in the UK. Retrieved from https://s4.chorus-mk.thirdlight.com/file/1573224908/63117952292/width=-1/height=-1/format=-1/fit=scale/t=444295/e=never/k=da5c189a/LeftStranded%20Report.pdf

Pearson, A., Rose, K. & Rees, J. (2023). 'I felt like I deserved it because I was autistic': understanding the impact of interpersonal victimisation in the lives of autistic people. Autism, 27(2), 500–511. https://doi.org/10.1177/13623613221104546

Ramachandran, V. S. (1980.) Introduction. In B. D. Josephson & V. S. Ramachandran (eds), *Consciousness and the Physical World: Edited Proceedings of an Interdisciplinary Symposium on Consciousness Held at the University of Cambridge in January 1978* (pp. 1–16). Pergamon Press.

Reza Arasteh, A. (1988). *Growth to Selfhood, The Sufi Contribution.* Routledge & Kegan Paul.

Varela, F. J., Maturana, H. R. & Uribe, R. (1974). Autopoiesis: the organisation of living systems, its characterization and a model. BioSystems, 5(4), 187–196.

Varela, F. J., Thompson, E. & Rosch, E. (1991). *The Embodied Mind: Cognitive Science and Human Experience.* MIT Press.

CHAPTER 8

Neurodiversity

Although Judy Singer wasn't the first to coin the term neurodiversity, her descriptions are clear: 'A biological truism that refers to the limitless variability of human nervous systems on the planet, in which no two can ever be exactly alike due to the influence of environmental factors' (Singer, 2020).

Neurodiversity is a concept that acknowledges and celebrates the natural variation in neurological differences among individuals. It emphasises that neurological conditions such as autism, ADHD, dyslexia, and others are part of the normal spectrum of human diversity, rather than being viewed as deficits or disorders. The neurodiversity movement seeks to challenge the medical model of disability and promote acceptance, inclusion, and accommodation for neurodivergent individuals. In 2024 an international group of autistic scholars of autism and neurodiversity showed that the concept and theory of neurodiversity, although previously primarily attributed to one person, Judy Singer, in fact has multiple, collective origins including from online communities of autistic people (Botha et al., 2024). It is important to correctly attribute this term to those who developed it.

The concept of autism as part of neurodiversity, akin to biodiversity, promotes a strengths-based difference model over a deficits-based medical model, emphasising the societal and individual benefits of fostering positive autistic identities, which can enhance self-esteem and improve mental health outcomes for autistic individuals (Cooper, Smith & Russell, 2017).

Fundamentally speaking, neurodiversity doesn't mean anything other than the difference between people. You can't say 'Jonny is neurodiverse'. You can't really even say 'Jonny is neurodivergent'. What or who does Jonny diverge from, exactly? But what else can we do with language? It's slippery stuff …

NEURODIVERSITY PARADIGM AND INTERSECTIONALITY, IN A YORKSHIRE ACCENT

So, you'll've 'eard t' word be now, neurodiversity an' as it says 'ere, it refers t' virtually infinite neurocognitive variability wi'in t'Earth's 'uman population. Everybody's gorra unique nervous system wi' a unique combination o' abilities an' needs.

If y'think abaht flowers, they's all sorts o' flowers an animals, an' subsets, it's same wi' neurology, an' folk, an' types, an' identities. Some are similar t'others, an collected together in diff'rent ways, but none of 'em are less than are they, that just dun't mek sense in t' biodiversity paradigm. It's all a complete whole, y'know? It's a feature o' t'Earth's biosphere. An 'ere we all are.

Think abaht t' infinite range o' differences in t'brain function, be'avioural traits, cognition – an' all of 'em 'ave evolved in response t' neuronormative assumptions. T' neurodiversity movement 'as come abaht as a response t' that, specially in context o' t'autistic spectrum, which, as you and I well know, is arguably t' most complex concept o' neurodiversity, reyt?

How did it feel when you read that? At home (if you're from Yorkshire)? Amused? Confused? Different? Alien? Othered?

It's just another accent. Why would someone who speaks differently to you or in a minority group be perceived as less than you? In Yorkshire, or supposing there was a bus full of Yorkshire people at the seaside in Brighton, the perspective ratio is contextual and dynamic too. It depends on who is in the majority and who is in the minority in different contexts.

PROBLEMS WITH NEURODIVERSITY

> While it is primarily a social justice movement, neurodiversity research and education is increasingly important in how clinicians view and address certain disabilities and neurological conditions.
>
> *(Baumer & Frueh, 2021, para. 2)*

In the neurodiversity paradigm, accommodations and compassion are being justified morally by modern society because of someone's deficits and weaknesses as per their unique brain. But ontologically, neurodiversity doesn't make sense. There's no reason to accommodate people who are simply just different. We should all accommodate each other.

Erin Manning is concerned with the philosophical problems of neurodiversity, in that it frames differences 'from the angle of typicality (divergence from the norm) and we see this difference as tied to a person, rather than seeing it as a mode' (Manning & Bozalek, 2024, p. 1).

This is an ongoing dialogue; my story, your story; all our stories coming together. Autism is the ideal focus for dialogue because of our relationship with the self (and what is the self?). Autism is from the word 'Autos', meaning 'self'. And there are some serious global concerns about the stability of ourselves as humans, neurodiversity, many other types of diversity and the human biosphere.

All 'neurotypes' are to be accepted as a natural part of our genetic legacy. In a way, there is only neurodiversity or neuroatypicality. All autistic people and all those with related 'neurodivergent' spectrum conditions such as Tourette's syndrome, dyslexia etc. are already fully accepted as equally important to our collective human evolution. Autism, a broad spectrum encompassing a large portion of neurodiversity, is the ideal focus for Dialogue; not only because of a perceived growing disparity between viewpoints (and a growing feeling among autistic and neurodivergent people who feel unrepresented and overlooked in society and research) but because of serious global concerns to the stability of the human biosphere. Autistic people are everywhere. Autism is everywhere. People are everywhere.

Exercise

Some questions you could ponder:

- What could Dialogue contribute to neurodiversity as a concept?
- How does using Dialogue acknowledge neurodiversity better or differently than other approaches?
- What is it about Dialogue that makes it a good way of interacting that avoids some of the problems people belonging to multiple marginalised groups experience in other settings and contexts?
- What is the neurodivergent diverging from?
- What is your thinking diverging from?

Dialogue practitioners and facilitators need to understand and work with the concept of unity in diversity and be sensitive to neurodivergent perspectives, including their own. Many educators, coaches and therapists don't even have training in the neurodiversity paradigm or autism awareness.

The healthcare professions especially should resist default normalisation. Disability is a dynamic and contextual social construction and not something solely within an individual so, therapists need to cultivate a relational humility regarding different experiences of neurodivergence, complex overlaps of intersecting categories of (minority) differences and disablement (Chapman & Botha, 2023). Dysfunction needs to be re-conceptualised as relational rather than individual. In other words, recognise what you don't know.

DOES THE NEURODIVERSITY PARADIGM COMPARE TO AUTISTIC GESTALT PROCESSING?

Neurodiversity shares common ground with autistic gestalt processing as they both emphasise different modes of thinking and perceiving the world, but focus on different scales of human experience. Neurodiversity stresses inclusivity, honouring the full range of mental experiences without pathology. Autistic gestalt processing is a specific cognitive style where, rather than processing information in a linear, step-by-step manner, the tendency is to take in large amounts of information at once, focusing on the whole rather than the details first. This 'big picture' or holistic thinking style may mean autistics perceive diverse patterns, connections, or nuances that others do not.

Perhaps in this way, everyone's ground of consciousness or 'pre-thought' is an ecology before it becomes an object. Bohm's (1980) 'rheo-mode' proposal for a language that emphasises the verb over the noun reflects Manning (n.d.), who proposes 'an ecological politics where movement and relation take precedence over predefined categories, such as the neurotypical and the neurodiverse, or the human and the nonhuman'.

This can also impact how autistic people understand language, for example, understanding phrases or expressions as whole units rather than breaking them into individual words. Echolalia is a function of the brain, which might be attempting to assimilate by repetition, and research is trending towards considering echolalia a developmental phenomenon in children's normal cognitive and linguistic maturation (Xie et al., 2023).

Using this example, we could assume that the neurodiversity paradigm or 'movement' is a way that the predominant 'neurotypical' human mind has conveniently manifested, in order to describe 'everyone' in a reductive, 'non-gestalt' way. Is it possible that 'neurotypical' people do not 'see the bigger picture' (as in autistic gestalt) and therefore created 'neurodiversity' as a reductive concept to explain diversity groupings, while autistic people already see the bigger picture and the idea of 'neurodiversity', which basically means everyone is different, is blindingly obvious? The implications of this are interesting.

Let's look at this some more. Autistic gestalt processing highlights that there isn't one 'correct' way to think and gestalt processing allows some autistic people to excel in areas like pattern recognition or systems thinking, so a holistic perspective offers advantages.

Neurodiversity as a concept takes a broad, inclusive view of human cognition, while gestalt processing takes a holistic approach to individual information processing. While both challenge reductionist approaches that attempt to break down or 'fix' ways of thinking into smaller, conventional parts, neurodiversity would seem akin to using a sledgehammer to crack a nut, indicating a perpetual fragmentation of society, which Bohm teaches us about. Bohm and Jenks (1994, p. 5) describe the phenomenon thus: 'Thought is participating and then saying it's not participating. But it is taking part in everything. Fragmentation is a particular case of that. Thought is creating divisions out of itself and then saying that they are there naturally'.

SO DO WE NEED NEURODIVERSITY AND, IF SO, WHY?

Neurodiversity opens up a spectrum where cognitive experiences are fluid and adaptable. Similarly, autistic gestalt processing may involve understanding meaning fluidly, with autistic people perhaps interpreting language or concepts in ways that are richer or more interconnected than neurotypical linear processing would allow.

In essence, autistic gestalt processing can be viewed as one manifestation of the neurodiverse spectrum, showing how unique cognitive styles exist within a broader, pluralistic understanding of mind and behaviour.

We move through a world in never-ending conversation with itself. It begins with a spark: an event, a phenomenon, a signal. Trees, responding to an infestation, produce insecticidal chemicals and exchange them across a network of roots. A predator ignites a murmuration of starlings, and each bird is simultaneously attracted to, repelled by, and in alignment with its neighbour, creating a perpetuating, liquid swirl. If we look at the sensing, processing, and exchanging of information happening in these situations, we can begin to see each as systems engaged in dialogue.

(Holt, 2019, p. 105)

REFERENCES

Baumer, N. & Frueh, J. (2021). What is neurodiversity? Retrieved from www.health.harvard.edu/blog/what-is-neurodiversity-202111232645

Bohm, D. (1980). *Wholeness and the implicate order.* Routledge & Kegan Paul.

Bohm, D., Jenks, C. (2004). *Thought as a System.* Taylor & Francis.

Botha, M., Chapman, R., Onaiwu, M. G., Kapp, S., Ashley, A. S., Walker, N. (2024). The neurodiversity concept was developed collectively: an overdue correction on the origins of neurodiversity theory. Autism, 28(6), 1591–1594. https://doi.org/10.1177/13623613241237871

Chapman, R., & Botha, M. (2023). Neurodivergence-informed therapy. Dev Med Child Neurol., 65(3), 310–317. https://doi.org/10.1111/dmcn.15384

Cooper, K., Smith, L. G. E., & Russell, A. (2017). Social identity, self-esteem, and mental health in autism. European Journal of Social Psychology, 47(7), 844–854. https://doi.org/10.1002/ejsp.2297

Holt, A. (2019). The conversation: feedback structures, ways of knowing, and neurodivergence. Public, *30*(59), 104–112. https://doi.org/10.1386/public.30.59.104_1

Manning, E. (n.d.). Erin Manning books. Retrieved from http://erinmovement.com/books

Manning, E., & Bozalek, V. G. (2024). In conversation with Erin Manning: a refusal of neurotypicality through attunements to learning otherwise. *Qualitative Inquiry*, online ahead of print. https://doi.org/10.1177/10778004241254397

Singer, J. (2020). Explaining neurodiversity. Retrieved from https://neurodiversity2.blogspot.com/2020/08/neurodiversity-what-it-is-and-isnt.html

Xie, F., Pascual, E., & Oakley, T. (2023). Functional echolalia in autism speech: verbal formulae and repeated prior utterances as communicative and cognitive strategies. Frontiers in Psychology, *14*, 1010615. https://doi.org/10.3389/fpsyg.2023.1010615

CHAPTER 9

Autism Dialogue and mindfulness

A mindful awareness model should be a core element of any client-helper interactions, not just an add-on. This chapter provides an introduction to a short programme I devised called Mindfulness for Autism (M4A), a core component of the Autism Dialogue Approach. M4A attempts to address some of the most prominent concerns in autistic interactions using specially adapted Mindfulness approaches, including cross-neurotype empathy and power, alternative and augmented communication, sensory sensitivities, complex trauma, vagal healing, self-care and compassion, masking and autistic/ADHD empowerment.

Mindfulness has become synonymous with huge programmes on a global scale but in simple terms mindfulness as a concept is 'learning to pay attention moment by moment, intentionally and with curiosity and compassion' (Kabat-Zinn, 2004), which we all knew very well how to do, before we forgot.

Low-level trauma can create a split between the psyche and the spirit, leading to emotional fragmentation and disconnection (Pec et al., 2014).

Exercise

Consider a low-level trauma or ongoing stressor you've experienced and how this has affected your sense of self and connection to your deeper essence.

Take a few conscious breaths and a moment of quiet.

Mindfulness for autism means reduced anxiety and stress, empowerment and developed identity among parents and academics and gives healthcare professionals a better understanding, leading to more cross-cultural cohesion. In Dialogue, by considering the power of a silent meditative approach, one can observe the movement of thought and language. Silence is an implicit and equally important part of the practice of communicating. In a constructive and safe environment, with plenty of quiet and silence, collective sense-making is more coherent, and common challenges typical in autism, such as sensory overload from noisy and busy environments, are addressed.

Extending into wider definitions of the environment, Bohm suggested exploring the roots of the many crises that face humanity today (Bohm, Factor & Garrett, 1991). As outlined in the initial parts of this book, my focus on autism and autos/self stems from a lifelong search for meaning and selfhood, and the need for a calmer, less fragmented life. I've been meditating in various ways since I was a child in the 1970s and spent much of my life inside spiritual communities. I know through experience that meditation practice can support and frame the search for belonging and inclusion and complement any life, spiritual or not. My personal position on creation, life, God, the universe, spirituality or unity consciousness is somewhat irrelevant and misses the point, when I'm introducing mind-clearing, relaxation and thought-attention in a Dialogue or individual coaching session. The same goes for systemic group coaching or delivering a mindfulness course with company executives – it's the ethics, relationships and holistic outcomes that matter.

As a regular solo practice, the benefits of mindfulness meditation are an antidote to stresses and strains, isolation, confusion and fragmentation and therefore must be hugely beneficial in autism.

If professional communication environments are to be truly participatory and ethical, allowing for genuinely collaborative sense-making, mindfulness, or mindful awareness is vital.

Mindfulness has become an overused term, so I use it here loosely to cover mindful awareness or meditation – which is a crucial element to successful autism dialogue and meaningful interconnectedness. I go further into this in Chapter 13 on Insight Dialogue, a framework that shares much of the ethos and activities with ADA.

INTRODUCTION TO MINDFULNESS

Modern mindfulness-based programmes are based on the Buddhist traditions of mindfulness meditation and adjusted to mental health care based on the Western science of psychology. It has become so widespread in the West that I recently heard Buddhist monks in Tibet are now learning from Western books on meditation. Mindfulness is described as present moment, non-judgmental awareness and may or may not use body or breath awareness as an 'anchor' to present moment experience, as we learn to watch the 'wandering mind'. Meditation is natural, it is 'resting in' who you are, so with that intention, we are resetting the dial for our real self, which can be described as calm and confidently perceptive. Mindfulness is a process, a practice to live by, so it might be difficult and feel like it's not working at first, but it is. You can see it as a practice where the more you do it the better you get. If you can persist, the results may be subtle at first, perhaps with occasional glimpses of deeper clarity or satisfaction. This might even be puzzling and even after years of practice, I still sometimes forget why I might be feeling strangely elevated, even though I may have just been to a new meditation group the day before, for example (this really just happened).

The benefits are physiological in that regular practice strengthens the immune system, helps relieve stress and anxiety, reduces chronic pain, alleviates depression and improves sleep. On the mental, emotional and spiritual levels, there are improved moods and fewer swings, improved empowerment, enhanced creativity, more peace of mind, more fun and happiness and (crucially for dialogue) better relationships. So meditation, together in groups or alone can be an antidote to stresses and strains, isolation, confusion and fragmentation.

Framing the search for deeper meaning in our lives with a thing we've called mindfulness can be extremely helpful and satisfying, and can complement any life, spiritual or not. Of course, there have always been many kinds of meditation everywhere, it's just that in the modern age, especially in the West, we appear to have lost our spiritual, communal roots to instead focus on information accumulation, positive knowledge, reductionist sciences, space travel, entertainment, escapism, individualism and consumerism. If that sounds bleak or exaggerated, take a moment to think about the modern cities we live in. Much of the negative impacts upon autistic people is because of the fast-paced, desensitised modern environments and the hegemony of the predominant neurotype. It seems like there's a problem with real communication.

SILENCE

Silence allows room for each person to process experiences in their own way, without pressure to conform to typical patterns of thought or behaviour. In silence, there's no 'right' way to be – each person's internal landscape is allowed to unfold at its own pace.

There are deeply transformative aspects to silence. Depending on your environment, imagine silence as something alive and present, filling the space, and infusing our feelings, thoughts and bodies. Imagine the richness and power of silence, not as an absence but as an active force that can transform and heal. How does silence feel for you, right now, in your body and mind? Does it bring a sense of calm, or does it heighten certain sensations? Pay attention to the diversity of your internal experience, without judgement. Invite silence into Dialogue.

We may ponder on a mysterious line between silence and sound. Like the edge of dawn where night meets day, it feels delicate and profound. Silence isn't merely the absence of sound – it's a space that holds sound, cradling it gently before it emerges or after it fades away. It's the breath before speech, the stillness that precedes music, the pause that gives rhythm its meaning. In silence, we are drawn to listen more deeply, to hear not just the external world, but the subtle sounds of our inner landscape. On this line, silence becomes a gateway, inviting us into the unknown, where sound begins to take shape. It's a place of potential, where the unsaid lingers, where our inner voices, thoughts, and even the heartbeat of the world around us can be heard most clearly.

Wayne Dyer puts it like this: 'Everything that's created comes out of silence. Your thoughts emerge from the nothingness of silence. Your words come out of this void. Your very essence emerged from emptiness. All creativity requires some stillness' (Dyer, 2004, p. 6). Did you see how he slips from silence to void to stillness?

With meditation we can discover the nature of the mind and the stress and suffering it causes and instead cultivate kindness, joy and compassion for ourselves and others; we can even create unshakeable inner peace and experience deep ecstatic union with the universe. Life can be a rough ocean with constant ups and downs, rolls and churning and with autistic lives, this is even more true. With meditation, anyone can dive below the surface of life, to where the water is calmer and more beautiful. With meditation, you will get to see the world where meditators have lived and benefitted for thousands of years.

While meditation can't promise to directly solve the external issues in your life, it will help you balance, develop inner resilience, and have the strength to keep up with challenges in life and find creative solutions. It can change the way you think, behave and respond to the world for your benefit. Even spending just ten minutes a day meditating, you'll develop new habits and responses and programme your system to experience better emotions and mind-states.

MINDFUL TALKING AND AWARENESS IN DIALOGUE GROUPS

Mindfulness works better with support. A regular meeting with a group will strengthen your community spirit, which is also crucial to stay healthy and happy. The New Economics Foundation carried out a global meta-analysis on healthy living and found connecting with others is the best way of staying healthy (Aked et al., 2008). It seems a long time since a lot of us knew what community really is, let alone sincere and meaningful communication. When was the last time you had what you would call a true sharing with your neighbour, even for a few minutes?

Before we discuss why mindfulness is useful for dialogue, let's look at some of the more common practices and principles.

We can have the intention to become aware of any of our particular senses. As we know they are seeing, smelling, tasting, hearing, and touching and we include a sixth sense – mental phenomena or thoughts and emotions. For example, being aware of emotions like sadness or love, or being aware of even basic thoughts and feelings.

Mindful yoga, exercise, tai-chi, chi gong or just looking, all result in the release of tension, stress and emotional trauma. You can really practise mindfulness anywhere, whether you're sitting, standing, running, lying down, swimming, when you're working around the house or out for a walk – and talking.

In the context of dialogue, we must first remember that all human life has great potential for meaning and joy. All notions of me, you, them, us – and autism – all are evolving constructs and not fixed. All of us are agents in regenerative systems (living, breathing human beings) and we can support and improve our healing and life-giving practices. In dialogic communities, we should be mindful of relational care and our responsibility to the whole. Autism, trauma and neurodiversity are paradigms to be explored through relationship-centred, proactive, caring and social justice approaches. Autism is therefore seen not as a tragedy or deficiency but as an opportunity for us to learn. If there is any agenda in a dialogue, it should be of generosity and compassion, because only if these human and spiritual foundations are allowed, will learning and change occur. Remember that autistic trauma is everyone's responsibility, and neurodiversity means all humans.

Autism dialogue is about working with each other. This connection to the 'other' neurotype is vital – we can't have one without the other – this is the dual becoming non-dual, like the Yin and Yang – the union of opposites. This more unified field of experience relates to autistic perception in the way Erin Manning (2018) describes it as 'a deep sensitivity to the coming-into-itself of form in experience'. Mindfulness means being aware of yourself in relation to others, whether that other is a person, animal, plant or thing. It is a shared energy exchange. If we can be more open to what Buber (2008) describes as the 'sacred space', this extra level of mindful awareness makes you more open to the other, yourself AND the relationship.

Insight Dialogue, which I cover in chapter 14, is a framework for deeply reflecting with another person, to relate to each other mindfully in the 'here and now'.

Suggested questions for mindfulness in dialogue

- What is 'relating mindfully'?
- Have you carefully considered all the different neurotypes in your group?
- Are you aware of your cross-neurotype experiences at work, home and in public places?
- What is the authentic self? Ask yourself when alone, then with ones you trust in dialogue.

SOME THOUGHTS ON SELF-ACCEPTANCE

Unmasking with others takes self-awareness, self-care and self-compassion.

Notice the alternating between you as the individual and you in a relationship with others. This is what the dharma (Buddhism), fellowship (Christianity) and ummah (Islam) teaches. It's why community is so important in living a life of mindful awareness.

Remember in autism we need to be even more sensitive about this due to the constraints and systemic trauma in pressure to conform. The lotus flower only grows in mud, and for this reason it is symbolic of the human condition. We can thrive in the worst situations.

Ask yourself what feelings there are inside.

Ask 'What do I feel?' or 'What do I want to think about that makes me feel?'

This is being intentional in mindfulness. In a way we can also choose but our feelings aren't usually controllable. There are so many distractions to avoid confronting our suffering. There's even a common habit of not even allowing good feelings to be fully experienced or last long, ideas that 'I am not worth it' or 'I don't deserve these feelings', the deep and wonderful feelings and emotions that are blocked from us really experiencing them.

Deep emotions are human emotions. We are afraid of being overwhelmed by true emotion but instead we are overwhelmed by thoughts. There is a saying that people used to laugh and cry more. We have become desensitised to our true feelings in the modern world with all its distractions and many people are stressed, unhappy and mentally ill. We are distracted and anxious, we are even anxious about feeling anxious, many people live in these negative cycles throughout their lives.

Listening exercise

To mindfully raise your hearing sensitivity,

Close your eyes. Take a few slow breaths and ask yourself, what are three things I can hear? Listen like you've never listened before.

Call a friend or (calm) family member on the phone. You might like to inform them what you want to do so you can share. Notice the tone of their voice, and be purposeful about truly listening to their words. Take five-minute turns to describe to each other what's happening in the moment. If you have a non-autistic or autistic friend – see what the differences are for you both.

INTEROCEPTION

Interoception is the inner relationship to one's own bodily experience. 'Interoceptive accuracy' refers to an individual's ability to shift attention internally and accurately track their physiological state.

For example, in social interaction, the typical bodily response to an uncomfortable situation might be an increase in heart rate, which can be to enhance alertness (e.g. argue or walk away). These physiological changes may (or may not) be felt, and they may (or may not) generate affect, and this is common in autism. Interoceptive ability may facilitate social connection, one of the biggest causes of self-harm, suicide ideation, and suicide. And loneliness may suggest interoceptive dysregulation.

Dialogue provides a positive feedback loop. Once one's social life starts to 'feel right,' one can start to trust/rely on their interoceptive signals even more in order to learn from social affective experience.

Exercise

Feel your body and ask yourself, *'what is happening for me right now?'* The body is part of our ecology, so if we tune into its unique voice it can be used to inform us what is happening – and reframing this can mean we are empowered by it, even if it doesn't feel okay. This is awareness, and awareness is power.

EFFORTLESS EFFORT

Effortless effort is a term from Eastern philosophy which I heard many years ago, and often think about. I think it's about showing up in the first place, then letting what's happening simply take over. It's a paradox whereby efficiency and effectiveness come from a place of ease and natural flow rather than relentless striving. Once you're there, where you wanted to be, let go. Find that harmonious balance where effort and ease coexist, creating a space for optimal performance and wellbeing.

Deeper still, effortless effort integrates learned skills with intuitive action. It involves being fully present and aware, without overthinking or forcing. When you're deeply engaged in the present moment, actions emerge spontaneously and smoothly. For this, you have to know how to connect with what T. S. Eliot (1943) called the 'still point of the turning world'.

Exercise

Close your eyes if you want and spend a moment reflecting silently on effortless effort – and accept whatever else comes up.

Think about a recent task where you experienced effortless effort.

Or just feel into it now. What made or makes this task feel effortless? How can you apply this understanding to areas where you feel strained or disconnected? You can achieve mastery and presence with ease, aligning with natural flow rather than force. Effortless effort can be applied to everyday tasks and personal growth. Open your eyes and come back to your presence in your room. You're doing mindfulness.

MANTRAS, MOVING AND OTHER CREATIVE DEVICES

Ancient languages such as Arabic and Sanskrit have deeper phonetic values and highly rhythmic purity of vibration. Compare this with echolalia – the involuntary repetition of words or phrases common in autism, which comes under the idea of vocal stimming and is sometimes voluntary. Chanting is an important part of many traditions.

Exercise

Consider making your own mouth sounds, like eclectic mantras. Vocal stimming is a huge source of joy and regulation for many autistic people.

In sensory overwhelm the brain stops processing sensory information – so mindfully attending to your five senses can help to bring regulation and the reintroduction of processing of sensory information that has stopped.

Exercise

Try this next time you are walking slowly.

Focus for five minutes on each of these:

- Everything you see
- Everything you hear
- Everything you feel
- Everything you smell

Each time your mind wanders, try just focusing on each leg movement saying 'left, right, left ...' then focus on the sensations again.

SOME EVIDENCE

Recent science suggests mindfulness-based programmes can benefit autistic people.

In one study by Riderinkoff et al. (2018) it was found that a combined mindfulness-based program for children and their parents was beneficial for autistic adolescents. Forty-five autistic children were referred, aged from eight to 19 years old, and their parents participated. Repeated measures were made of children's and parents' social communication problems, emotional and behavioural functioning, mindful awareness, and of parenting. After a two-month follow-up, then a one-year follow-up, while children did not report significant changes in mindful awareness, their social communication problems decreased, and their emotional and behavioural functioning improved. Improvements reported by children were most substantial at a two-month follow-up. This suggests that autistic children, including adolescents and their parents, can benefit from a mindfulness-based program with parallel sessions for children and parents.

Executive functioning could be improved by training mindfulness, because it is practised to control the focus of attention, to flexibly shift attention, to reflect on experiences, and thereby to notice one's automatic impulses which enables responding with awareness instead of reacting impulsively (Zelazo & Lyons, 2012).

Another study by Gaigg et al. (2020) found that self-guided mindfulness and cognitive behavioural practices reduce anxiety in autistic adults. After a 3-month follow up over 75% of participants 'demonstrated reliable reductions in at least one of the anxiety measures. This research was published in the Autism Journal. It was supported by the City University of London and the Medical Research Council.

REFERENCES

Aked, J., Marks, N., Cordon, C. & Thompson, S. (2008). *Five Ways to Wellbeing: A Report Presented to the Foresight Project on Communicating the Evidence Base for Improving People's Well-being*. New Economics Foundation. Retrieved from https://neweconomics.org/uploads/files/five-ways-to-wellbeing-1.pdf

Bohm, D., Factor, D. & Garrett, P. (1991). Dialogue – a proposal. Retrieved from https://aofpd.org/library/public-resources/dialogue-a-proposal/

Buber, M. (2008). *I and Thou*. Howard Books.

Dyer, W. (2004). *Wake Up ... Live the Life You Love, Finding Your Life's Passion*. Global Partnership.

Eliot, T. S. (1943). *Four Quartets*. Harcourt, Brace and Co.

Gaigg, S. B., et al. (2020). Self-guided mindfulness and cognitive behavioural practices reduce anxiety in autistic adults: a pilot 8-month waitlist-controlled trial of widely available online tools. *Autism*, 24(4), 867–883. https://doi.org/10.1177/1362361320909184

Kabat-Zinn, J. (2004). *Wherever You Go, There You Are*. Piatkus.

Manning, E. (2018). Histories of violence: neurodiversity and the policing of the norm. Retrieved from https://lareviewofbooks.org/article/histories-of-violence-neurodiversity-and-the-policing-of-the-norm

Pec, O., Bob, P. & Raboch, J. (2014). Splitting in schizophrenia and borderline personality disorder. *PLoS One*, 9(3), e91228. doi: 10.1371/journal.pone.0091228.

Ridderinkhof, A., de Bruin, E. I., Blom, R. & Bögels, S. M. (2018). Mindfulness-based program for children with autism spectrum disorder and their parents: direct and long-term improvements. *Mindfulness*, 9(3), 773–791. https://doi.org/10.1007%2Fs12671-017-0815-x

Zelazo, P. D. & Lyons, K. E. (2012). The potential benefits of mindfulness training in early childhood: a developmental social cognitive neuroscience perspective. *Child Development Perspectives*, 6(2), 154–160. https://doi.org/10.1111/j.1750-8606.2012.00241.x

CHAPTER 10

Guide to hosting an Autism Dialogue

In an Autism Dialogue session, participants engage in structured, reflective conversations designed to improve understanding, connection, and self-expression among autistic people, their supporters, and others. The focus is on creating a safe, inclusive space where everyone can contribute in their own way without judgement or pressure to conform to neurotypical communication norms. Participants focus on presence, active listening, and honouring diverse modes of expression.

For a full explanation of the four Dialogue practices, please see Chapter 5.

INTRODUCTION

Dialogue as a practice is simple and easy to learn because it's the most natural way of communicating in a group. In a way, you can't 'get it wrong' because it's a human quality and in the shared space, the dialogue event, we're all moving together towards shared and collective thinking.

If someone doesn't feel like speaking in the group it's okay. Turning up is the hardest bit. Being there means you're taking part, even just by listening. On Zoom or other video platforms it's better if people can see each other because of the non-verbal cues we get from each other, but if they are not happy to have their camera on that's fine too.

In the group, there should be anywhere between 10 and 25 together. Any less than 10 starts to dissolve the energy and any more than 25 creates distractions and fragmentation.

Preferably, people will attend all of the sessions in a series and you might have three, six, ten or more over several weeks or months, which is better for growing familiarity, confidence and therefore insight, but demonstrates a commitment to the new and evolving community. As time progresses you will all grow together and learn together more, and there's the opportunity to make friends and network.

HOW TO PREPARE FOR A DIALOGUE

A lot of good facilitation and reducing possibilities of anxieties arising will be in your preparation. Some practical approaches might include:

- What are your own support mechanisms and who are you working with?
- Provide information in advance in different forms.
- Enable communication of the other senses and other methods.
- Think about Augmented/assistive and Alternative Communication (AAC).
- Create appropriate visuals for co-designed 'ground rules'.
- Talking is taken for granted so think about Zoom where visual communication is limited.

Think about echolalia which is the spontaneous repetition of all or part of sentences, as a verbal response (Patra & De Jesus, 2023). Vocal stimming – self-stimulatory exercises with the mouth and vocal cords such as singing, clicking and tics (relates to Tourette's).

- Alexithymia is when a person has difficulty experiencing, identifying, and expressing emotions – so think about the implications of this when asking others about how they feel. Alexithymia commonly co-occurs with certain mental health conditions, including depression and post-traumatic stress disorder (PTSD) (Putica et al., 2023).

Facilitators having training in interpersonal methods (and being able to challenge such training from an autistic perspective) is almost vital, so is creating a structure of support around you.

Who's invited, who isn't?

I've grappled with questions like, 'Who am I inviting into the dialogue?' and 'What influences my decision to invite certain people?' While facilitating a Dialogue, I sometimes wonder if I've 'curated' a diverse group that reflects the local community, such as autistic individuals, perhaps one who's unemployed, a researcher, a teacher, or a parent, and I wonder about race and gender balances. Too often I wonder why there are no Black or Asian people or autistic non-speakers. Sometimes, I've had the unsettling feeling that the group is unintentionally speaking on behalf of autistic people who can't or don't speak, or those who might not leave their homes often. In these situations, we expose the fragmentation that exists within our communities and ourselves. It's not easy work, but it's necessary to push ourselves through these uncomfortable spaces to truly grapple with the complexities of identity, power, and representation. I heard a saying about dialogue once, that 'whoever turns up are the right people', which helps when I remember it.

A conducive environment for Dialogue

This is by no means a comprehensive list and one must remain aware, not just that all autistic people are different (what does 'autism-friendly' even mean?), but an autistic-non-autistic gathering will always be very dynamic.

The venue

If you have hired a room you need to visit and get to know it and the staff well. Think about any issues that could lead to confusion over, for example, venue directions, parking, entrance, reception staff, times etc. You could also see if there's a quiet space if anyone needs time out on their own for a short time. A photo of the venue entrance and the actual room can be extremely helpful in reducing pre-meeting nerves. Could you go that extra step to ask anyone if anyone has any special requirements or communication preferences?

Keep it simple for inclusivity

Once in your dialogue, before discussing the space with participants (which is a good thing to do), consider that clarity and simplicity in the meetings are important, to avoid any confusion about practicalities. You will want to consider all equal opportunities for dialogue contributions.

You could say a few things at the beginning to indicate acceptance and an inclusive ethos, so this would mean explaining that anyone is free to wander or leave without saying anything. Some autistic people might love to hear they're being thought about but without being singled out. Making sure someone's OK (particularly if you think they might not be) means you might have to ask them tactfully. This can mean extra pressure for the facilitator and co-facilitator/organiser but more inclusivity and participation means you'll get a wider and more representational range of voices, so that could mean engagement from more sensitive autistic people.

Sensory environment

A reminder about autistic people's ability to effectively engage socially will be affected by sensory stimuli in the environment, such as smells (e.g. strong perfume), noise (e.g. ticking clocks, phones, printers, roadworks) and light (e.g. if the sun is in someone's eyes they may not feel socially confident enough to say so). Bright lights (especially office strip lights) nearly always have a negative effect on an autistic person. Be aware of one person pointing at someone else or using a dominant voice often found in debates (especially talking over others or for a long time), this can be overwhelming for an autistic person. An autistic person might not be able to report, demonstrate or modulate anxiety. Anxiety is often addressed by self-silencing (muting), which can make things worse for them.

Boundaries

Keep a watch on boundaries in the community. People might know each other. Working with everyone (rather than to, for or on…). Being an ally, whether you are autistic or not, is crucial.

Be specific around timing. Your dialogue could be anywhere from an hour to a full day. An announced five-minute break should literally be a five minute break and at the exact time stated.

Keep an eye on possible interruptions – there's nothing worse than someone coming in the room at a highly charged moment because they forgot their umbrella (also relates to sensory input).

Interruptions can come from an individual. See below for an example of what happened when someone resisted being in a dialogue because of misunderstanding (boundaries and contracting).

Splitting into small groups for a workshop activity could be fine if you and the others want to and there are clear instructions and guidance (but not over-elaborated either). Nothing is ever compulsory. Sometimes a 'round table discussion' is useful but male sure there is plenty of space at each place – a 'hole in the middle' table format means more space and less sensory risk in your autism-friendly environment (smells, gaze, loud voices etc.). However, I've never done this because it creates a barrier.

Stimming

Stimming is becoming more common in public, so for example, someone might need a hand-pressure squeeze tool to modulate their senses if they need it. Someone might also wiggle their feet or hands a bit or doodle. Any repetitive motion is either automatic or intentional, in order to modulate sensory input, but can also be a sign of increased anxiety (Kapp et al., 2019). Someone used to bring a bag of stim toys and share them, which is great if they are clean.

Triggers

An important aspect to consider is a 'trigger', i.e. sensitive information spoken can trigger responses – here is where excellent facilitation is needed for maintaining the safe environment. An agreed practice can be saying 'trigger warning' or 'content warning' at the beginning of a delivery containing sensitive, emotion-inducing information (e.g. abuse or suicide) is good practice. Asking people to practice checking their conscience before speaking is good i.e. 'How does it feel if I imagine sharing that now?'

LET'S BEGIN!

Contracting

Contracting is crucial to bring right into the room with you, up front. It is a term borrowed from coaching and although group Dialogue isn't coaching it shares some of the same principles and ethos. The contract is your co-designed, working, dynamic agreement and belongs to everyone; you all agree to it and stick to it. When something is in doubt it's the first place you go and if you see something's missing, you put it on it.

Contracting covers all the processes for setting up the relationship. Typically in coaching, these include getting to know each other, establishing the grounds for relationship success, creating and maintaining rapport, and clarifying mutual expectations within the relationship. Transpose these principles into inviting participants to Dialogue. The key to safe and sound contracting is to set the agreement in advance and keep it alive. Always refer back to the contract and regularly re-contract if you need to.

Contracting content suggestions

- Essentials – (clarity of comms, numbers, venue, booking, cancellations, liability, etc.).
- Confidential reporting and note-taking.
- Reviews and evaluation/by whom/sharing of (see Appendix 1).
- Be very clear about times, breaks, frequency and how many sessions there are.
- Discuss everything openly and honestly.
- Review the relationships as you go.
- The participants may be reluctant to raise the subject of ending and emotionally affected (see below on closure).
- Do you feel you aren't achieving enough?
- Check the participants' support needs going forward.
- Review the contract regularly, refer to it always.
- Has a feedback form been co-designed?
- What are your own support mechanisms and who are you working with?

Whether it's the first session or not, it begins by laying out any co-contracting and setting clear ground rules to ensure psychological safety. As you meet each time elaborating decreases, but the basic minimum is always necessary.

Here's an example of something you might like to say, which you are free to adapt to your own purposes:

> Hello everyone. So … dialogue … here we all are.

Pause, relax and scan the room, allowing people to relax and to show you are comfortable with silence and what's arising.

> What is Dialogue? We might ask ourselves what we are thinking together, and what that means. This is a very basic idea of what real Dialogue aims to find out.
>
> What are we thinking – *together*?
>
> Dialogue is quite an unusual and radical form of communication.
>
> Our commonality here is also autism and its very many facets. Together we are a microcosm and we represent a small cross-section of the autism community (whatever that means to you). So whatever happens reflects the macrocosm,

our wider worlds ... We have come together in a unique and special way. Let's take a step back and remember why we have all come here.

Pause.

As we head into this session and remember why we are together, let's unpack our shared commonality a little more, together, to see more of where we are, what problems we face and together where we might hope to go.

As a reminder, Dialogue is not solution-focussed or support focussed, it is not for research or driven by any agenda. It is more of exploring together our 'sense of what is to come' in a conscious and caring environment. Dialogue serves as a safe container in which our community can think together. Initially, we need to literally talk about what this means – what is dialogue and why are we doing dialogue? Let's try and remain suspended in this question together and see how things feel. Yes?

Pause without expectation. If someone speaks, accept it and welcome it ... things are beginning to unfold.

We also need to encourage more questions to each other. Dialogue is also about what's not being said. Let's try to allow the space for *each other* to say what is not being said.'

Here the four practices and principles of dialogue can be read out if it doesn't sound repetitive teaching exercise. Perhaps everyone has seen them beforehand:

- Authenticity (finding one's own true voice).
- Listening (to what is really being said).
- Respect (ensuring things make sense to each other).
- Suspension (nurture enquiries into one's own thinking).

Additional guidelines

This could be part (or a repeat) of the contracting, depending on how you want to do it, and you might learn from getting it wrong, which is how things happen sometimes. There's a fine balance to strike with information and awareness. Beware of providing too much information and be prepared to switch attention to attending to each other – it might seem obvious but it's why you're all there!

- Speak slow enough and loud enough for everyone to hear, making sure you are understood.
- Please be sensitive and mention it before you speak about very sensitive issues (part of self-safeguarding) so others can be forewarned. Equally, speak up respectfully if you don't think something is appropriate. We all support each other within the dialogic practice and not attack.

- Confidentiality – everything said in the room stays in the room and identities are undisclosed outside the room.
- Identity first terminology is preferred by most 'autistic people'.
- No jargon or you may lose someone – be aware.
- There is no hierarchy. We all aim to facilitate.

Here are some points to consider for the session: shared goals will deepen awareness, increase participation, respect and a greater openness and sense of potential. Does it make sense? Do you agree – or not?

Some questions and thoughts to keep you going through the session:

- What is learned in dialogue and what really is dialogue and thinking together?
- Asking questions then asking where a question arose from is good practice.
- Notice the difference between thinking (now) and thought (past).
- What are we bringing and what exactly have we got to work with?
- Some discomfort is inevitable; this is part of the work.

We want to encourage everyone to speak in your own way – openly and authentically, while respecting the unique communication styles of others. Silence, slower pacing, and different ways of expressing ourselves, whether verbal, non-verbal or through gestures, are all welcomed.

Someone might start writing notes and hold them up (if they choose to, or if they go situationally mute). When this happens make sure everyone can read it – if not, offer (directly to the person) to read them out.

Two trained facilitators guide the session, helping participants stay focused and ensuring that everyone has the opportunity to contribute in their own way, even just by being present. (See chapter 11 on Facilitation Awareness). The role of the facilitator is not to direct the conversation but to create an environment where the dialogue can unfold naturally. They may invite participants to share experiences or reflections, encouraging open-ended discussion rather than rigid topics.

Participants practise active listening, where they focus fully on others' words and expressions without immediately responding or interpreting. This encourages a deeper level of engagement and reduces the pressure to respond quickly or in expected ways. Reflection is also emphasised, allowing participants to process what has been said before speaking.

Autism Dialogue sessions typically avoid traditional hierarchies. Instead of one person dominating the conversation, each participant is given equal space to share their thoughts, ensuring a balanced exchange. This structure encourages autistic individuals to feel valued for their perspectives, regardless of communication style.

The dialogue is centred on personal experience and shared reflection, rather than debate or persuasion. The goal is not to reach a consensus or solve problems but to explore different perspectives and gain a deeper understanding. Participants are encouraged to express their inner worlds, often in ways that may not be easily conveyed in more conventional dialogue.

Discussions often explore what it means to be autistic and how different people experience the world. This might, for example, include reflections on sensory processing, social interactions, self-identity, or challenges related to masking. Participants can share how their autistic traits shape their lives, both positively and negatively, fostering mutual understanding.

Periods of silence are an integral part of Autism Dialogue sessions. These moments allow participants to reflect and process the conversation without the pressure to fill the space with words. Silence is valued as much as speech, recognising that dialogue happens at different paces for different people.

Participants often gain new insights, not just into autism but also into communication, empathy, and human diversity. Both autistic and non-autistic participants can develop a deeper appreciation for each other's perspectives, leading to greater mutual understanding and connection. Autism Dialogue sessions aim to create a supportive, non-judgmental space for exploring experiences, fostering both individual and collective growth. They focus on presence, active listening, and honouring diverse modes of expression, making them a powerful tool for building connection and insight.

Ideas for checking in

Integral to Dialogue is some form of 'check-in'. There are endless ways to check in. I prefer the phrase 'warm-up' to 'ice-breaker' for obvious reasons, but we can still reflect on what it is that requires warming up.

You can begin with a dynamic little self-enquiry exercise to ascertain a sense of autonomy and equity among participants. Ask the group to ask themselves: 'Why are you here?' This will begin identifying desired outcomes and forming a sense of consensus and alignment. Conduct and expectations like 'confidentiality' and 'no interrupting' can be unanimous and agreed upon by participants at the outset via the check-in and collating these is one of the jobs of the facilitators. Incorporate more intersubjective energy as the session and programme unfolds, you can use the method of 'check-up' (part-way) and 'check-out' (at completion) as a type of self-scaling.

Once you've all checked in (or passed if someone doesn't want to) you need a starter theme. Ask: 'What is Autism?' or 'What is Dialogue?' and be prepared to launch but verbally state that the dialogue has begun – this is important for clear contracting. You might have to spend more than one or two sessions learning what Dialogue is, and unlearning what it isn't. Great, you're on your way!

How to address common themes

Sometimes the dialogue will hover around common themes such as sensory experiences. When you feel the conversation is doing this, don't automatically assume it's got stuck and try to move it on – this could be destructive to the flow. You need to hold the space, whatever happens – you are exactly what the dialogic system needs at that moment – a holder of space – the word facilitation means *to make it easier*.

All communication has aspects of sharing, performance and storytelling. As a facilitator, you need to be attuned to how this might change quickly back and forth, faster than a blink, between different people and in the same person. You may witness different kinds of trauma behaviour and potential for triggering – what do you do if someone is triggered?

A good question, so ask the group!

Some topics like death are too often taboo in society, so be prepared to have an honest dialogue, while being extra-sensitive to all participants. It could be useful to do a pause and quick check around the room. Or prepare the group, intervening with the words 'trigger warning here' if the conversation moves into these areas, including self-harm and suicide. In a community group, I wouldn't want to bring in suicide as it's too precarious and takes on a different level of awareness, implicit contracting and moves into mental health arena. This would be different from, say for example, a conversation about what happens after death, religious beliefs and interesting death-related experiences which don't involve threats to mental stability or group safety.

Have you thought about how you might deal with topics such as sex, emotions, drugs, addictions, and other disclosures? Sometimes facilitators learn from experience too.

'Spiritual experiences' may be had by participants, but this is not the aim. Feelings of heightened awareness, out of body, intense joy can be followed by fear, sadness, relief or other emotions. It is not the aim of Dialogue to work with or analyse an individual's experiences and certainly, therapeutic lines shouldn't be taken by anyone. The point of contracting is also to let people know what dialogue is not – and it isn't anything explicitly to do with therapy, breakthroughs, self-realisation or enlightenment. Participants are not clients and people who bring overtly personal or subjective healing or spiritual-type agendas should be checked, perhaps asking 'Is there anything you want to ask the group about that?' This is a subtle way to bring it back to 'the middle' and make the Dialogue relevant to everyone. Watch out for therapists and clients or people known to clients, especially in town and city communities. Dialogue supervision among a group of therapy students or practitioners is different.

Spirituality isn't an aim or a method or a practice in Dialogue, it certainly can't explicitly be applied to autism and if the facilitator attempts to do this, she risks fragmenting the group between those who 'know' and those who 'don't know.' Any reports of spiritual insights should be welcome as much as other reporting and held within the group's process. Ethical integrity for the facilitator is paramount.

WHEN BOUNDARIES AREN'T IN PLACE

What if someone at a Dialogue session says something like, 'Can you help me with my financial support application?' This really happened. They'd been 'referred' by another service and hadn't chosen to attend and therefore didn't really understand why they were there. I helped them gently in the group by asking if they know why they are here. (They were already there so I had to deal with it!) The person wasn't comfortable, so I had to use a backup plan and my co-facilitator invited that person into the lobby for a side-talk and they decided to leave. We followed up by email later and found out where the invitation breach lay.

Someone else once announced half way through a first session with a large group of mostly very sensitive people, 'This is just silent consensus.' (meaning they assumed there was a hidden agenda and weren't comfortable with that assumption). The group unpacked that a little, led by me, but it was quickly clear they hadn't understood what the method was and why they were there, continuing to push back in a way that was disruptive to the whole group's process. I was admittedly uncomfortable (which was obvious) and had to make a decision to preserve the whole group. At the break I asked the person a little bit more assertively if they were comfortable because, I said, they were making everyone else uncomfortable. They decided to leave. The group was saved and it showed me how sensitive and open everyone was. I learned lessons about clarity of contracting and thankfully this kind of thing hasn't happened again.

What would you have done?

CLOSURE

As a series of Autism Dialogue sessions draws to a close, it's essential to approach the transition with sensitivity, acknowledging the depth of connection and emotions participants may feel. For some, group intimacy might be a new and potentially unsettling experience, making it vital to create a space for open reflection. Facilitators can invite participants to share their feelings about the journey, ensuring everyone's voice is heard and validated. Emphasising the skills and insights gained, facilitators might encourage participants to carry forward these practices into their everyday lives. Offering gratitude for each person's contributions and reinforcing the sense of community built, facilitators can also provide resources or opportunities for ongoing connection, helping participants feel supported as they transition out of the group environment. There are many creative ways to sensitively close a series of dialogues and you can invent your own too.

RECORDING FEEDBACK

Have a feedback system as it's great for you knowing things worked or didn't.
Someone once wrote:

> I thoroughly enjoyed today's conversations, they flowed like a river, we were in a river and I was the river. Topics flowed like 'What is autism?', 'What autism means to me', 'The benefits and challenges associated with autism' and 'What can society do to improve lives for autistic people and their families?'. I feel washed with new meanings.
>
> *(Autism Dialogue community participant, personal communication, 2019)*

Enough things to think about.
It's time to start designing your programme.

REFERENCES

Kapp, S. K., Steward, R., Crane, L., Elliott, D., Elphick, C., Pellicano, E. & Russell, G. (2019). 'People should be allowed to do what they like': Autistic adults' views and experiences of stimming. *Autism*, 23(7), 1782–1792.

Patra, K. P. & De Jesus, O. (2023). Echolalia. Retrieved from www.ncbi.nlm.nih.gov/books/NBK565908/

Putica, A., Van Dam, N. T., Felmingham, K., Lawrence-Wood, E., McFarlane, A. & O'Donnell, M. (2023). Interactive relationship between alexithymia, psychological distress and posttraumatic stress disorder symptomology across time. *Cognition and Emotion*, 38(2), 232–244. https://doi.org/10.1080/02699931.2023.2283934

CHAPTER 11

Autism Dialogue facilitation skills

....

Whatever your reasons for running a series of Autism Dialogues in the community, it can be a highly charged yet very rewarding activity. The group can experience a certain transcendence and many people report a feeling of *koinonia* (spiritual fellowship) and deep insight and realisation, even spiritual experiences. I have noticed this among autistic or otherwise sensitive people.

Of course, this might be the last thing on the minds of a group of pressurised staff at a first meeting in a corporate environment, but if you're an executive group coach, I ask you to think again. I invite you to think outside the box. Let me rephrase that – I ask you to notice your feelings as you consider there never was or ever will be a box. So forget the box. A facilitator has to navigate the unknown realms of the unknown, in service of the group, its processes and its participants.

As a useful reference, take this description:

> They speak now through one mouth, now through another. Active currents within the group may be expressed or come to a head in one particular person, between particular persons, or may, in a sense, be 'personified' in individuals. But whatever is going on in the group is always regarded by us as a process developing in this total group.
>
> *(Foulkes & Anthony, 2018, p. 259)*

If you experience something like that in the boardroom, you're working at the right place.

Group dialogue processes can be time-consuming, which may not be ideal for fast-paced or urgent professional situations; this brings us to the point about context. Dialogues in organisations often involve extensive discussions and consensus-building, which can slow down decision-making processes. When not well-facilitated, group dialogue can devolve into unproductive debates or tangential discussions, wasting participants' time and hindering progress. In some group settings, certain individuals may dominate the conversation, while others remain passive. This can lead to unequal participation and may not reflect the full range of perspectives. People may have different levels of resistance to the idea of group dialogue, preferring more traditional hierarchical decision-making structures and viewing the facilitator as a teacher. Effective group dialogue requires skilled facilitation and a clear process. An autistic facilitator is essential, while having two might feel unbalanced. One of each (like socks) is good because it models the dynamic tensions in society – and it is crucial you both are familiar with each other and have good 'chemistry'.

Integrity before, during and after the group process is key to success and that's why many people report disappointment when a series comes to an end and they are faced with the fragmentation of wider society once more. During the dialogue process, without a level of ethical maturity, wisdom and integrity on the part of the facilitator and therefore the whole facilitation process, dialogues can become chaotic or unproductive, leading to frustration among participants. Group dialogue is not immune to bias and prejudice. If not properly managed, it can perpetuate existing power dynamics and reinforce stereotypes or discriminatory behaviours.

Group dialogue can be a valuable professional framework for fostering collaboration, problem-solving, and effective communication. However, it is not without its challenges, including potential inefficiency, resistance to change, and the need for skilled, sensitive but robust and wise facilitation.

PARTICIPATORY CONSIDERATIONS

True participation can never be underestimated and the main setting in which problems are being seen is where non-autistic people speak on behalf of autistic people, without due caution. The autistic community values the experience of being autistic. In an 'autism awareness' training environment, we seriously recommend you consider autistic person delivery, as the last thing you want is to alienate (or worse, distress) an autistic trainee with what is often seen as 'an outsider view'.

The National Autistic Society have a good introductory video called 'Make it Stop' (National Autistic Society, 2017).

The future is going to be more participatory, with autistic voices getting stronger. Everyone needs a basic understanding of autism and everyone can benefit from knowing how to create an autism-friendly environment. Just remember, the definition of a sensory or social environment is one consideration, and 'if you've met one autism-friendly environment you've met one autism-friendly environment!'

DIGITAL AGE

Online, the internet allows us to do our work easily and research shows autistic people in this context are comfortable using the internet for communication purposes (Benford & Standen, 2009). The connection between local and international beneficiaries is important to our development of perceived cultural differences in autism and building bridges globally will help build a conceptual framework for scaling while remaining fully aware of cultural differences here in the UK.

Modern communication breakdown and social fragmentation are complex phenomena influenced by various factors. The advent of the computer age and digital communication technologies has drastically changed the way we communicate. While these technologies have connected people across the globe (and provided our organisational networks with easy global access to each other, which may otherwise be prohibitive, and many successful dialogues and training sessions), they have also introduced new challenges. Digital communication often lacks the richness of face-to-face interaction, leading to a potential breakdown in meaningful communication (Newson et al., 2021).

In digital spaces like Zoom, we can connect across cultures and languages instantly, but communication challenges persist and without being physically present, we often experience a disconnect – missing the rich, embodied nuances of in-person interaction. Someone might say something important in the chat box, which pops up and interrupts the vocal conversation. Side chats take place, diluting the power of unified thinking, but turning it off can mean excluding those who aren't speaking so an example of keeping things accessible for all might be allowing participants to direct message a facilitator who can relay their words to the group. Emojis, slang, and abbreviations vary by community, culture, and generation, which, while often convenient, is open to widespread misunderstandings. This absence of physical cues can create a subtle, but impactful, barrier to fully connecting and communicating with one another in the way we would face-to-face.

When I used to hear of 'Zoom fatigue' from people in other groups, I noted this wasn't present in me or any of the participants in our lengthy (up to four hours) group dialogues online; in fact it was usually the opposite, with me and others present reporting a sense of being spiritually nourished and socially recharged. This demonstrates something about the quality of interpersonal contact and the setting up and maintaining of psychologically safe environments. There's a lot more to be explored about the difference between online and in-person group activities, something which came to the fore during the COVID lockdown periods of 2020–2022.

FACILITATING DIALOGUE: RESPONSIBILITY AND ETHICS

It is not the purpose of this book to attempt to provide comprehensive facilitator training. Facilitators serve as role models who embody and actively promote deep understanding, empathy, tolerance and respect, suspend assumptions and opinions and treat all people as equals. That said, please make sure your insurance is valid and you're wearing clean socks.

In our group work, two trained and experienced facilitators will make sure the group is moving along the right way; as mentioned previously, at least one of them needs to identify as autistic. If one is and one isn't and they work together well, this can model the dynamic of structural duplicity and provide not just an example but a model, and help increase trust. Their lived experience is valuable.

It is important to remember that the facilitator is never apart from the process. Good facilitation needs to support safety, equity and trust, without compromise. Facilitators guide participants from the first point of contact and are always available throughout the helping process. Once in the setting, they will 'hold the space' for participants, using a range of modalities and techniques, including some easy-to-learn practices, which are rooted and upheld by deep philosophical and spiritual values.

Facilitators should adhere to a set of professional standards and accreditations, such as those of the European Mentoring and Coaching Council (EMCC) and/or the British Association for Counsellors and Psychotherapists (BACP). There is not yet an association or council for Professional Dialogue, however, the Academy of Professional Dialogue (AoPD) has one under development. A truly dialogic approach is one of equal learning status where facilitators both learn and help generate insight and understanding. Learning together means creating empowerment, to make changes that are meaningful to the group, with the understanding and awareness of greater shared meaning.

ETHICAL CONSIDERATIONS

Ethical maturity is having the reflective, rational and emotional capacity to decide what is right and/or wrong, having the courage to do it and being accountable ethically for the decision (Carroll, 2011). All sorts of things are considered in professional dialogue and coaching, for example, competence, context, boundary management, integrity, one's own values (personal and professional), the development journey and limits of own competence, knowing when to refer on, clear and well thought through contracting, self-care, frankness, openness and honesty, self-care and contingencies such things go wrong.

EVALUATING DIALOGUE: THE ART OF NOT KNOWING AND NAVIGATING UNCERTAINTY

> Delusion arises when we are not sensitive to incoherence when we overlook it.
> *(David Bohm cited in Wijers, 1996, p. 62)*

> [U]ncertainty is deeply salient to hoping, not only because hope as a concept entails epistemic limits, but more vitally because not knowing, when done skillfully and when supported through education and some degree of socio-economic security, leaves room for others to reframe utterances, and so for the family or community to resist linguistic enclosure.
> *(Cuffari, Fourlas & Whatley, n.d., para. 1)*

The word evaluation is from the Latin *valere* ('to be strong, well, of value, of worth'). For me, there's an important question about social values' alignment with scientific evaluation. Dialogue as a research methodology in and of itself has some way to go. I'm not an academic and can't think beyond ideas of grounded theory, action research and interpretative phenomenological analysis; IPA is a qualitative research method that examines how people make sense of their experiences, and the meaning they attach to them – often used in the social sciences to study complex, ambiguous, or emotionally charged topics. Meanwhile, I suggest if you want to know if the Dialogue worked, ask the participants before and after, then get in touch with them sometime later to do a review. Ask them if their life satisfaction has improved.

FACILITATING THE GENERATIVE POTENTIAL OF DIALOGUE

Embodying and living according to the four dialogic practices (outlined in Chapter 6) will enhance our ability as facilitators to connect with others. When applied well by example, they can enhance collective sense-making and everyone's ability to participate on a deeper level.

Connecting with the possibility for something new, creative, or transformative to emerge from a situation, interaction, or process is referred to as generative potential. Attuning to the process of generative potential, the underlying energy or force that gives rise to growth, innovation, and positive change is the central role of the facilitator. This means he or she must be always aware of the deeper currents of creativity, connection, and understanding that can arise, especially when participants are truly present, open, and engaged with one another.

The term is often used in contexts like dialogue, creativity, systems thinking, and leadership to describe the fertile ground from which new ideas, insights, or solutions can emerge.

In practical terms, generative potential involves various elements:

- Creativity: The possibility for original or innovative ideas to surface in a given space or conversation.
- Transformation: The ability of an individual, group, or system to undergo meaningful change or growth.
- Emergence: A dynamic, evolving process where something new and previously unseen comes into being as a result of interactions, openness, or collaboration.
- Connection and Synergy: This arises when people, ideas, or forces come together in such a way that the sum is greater than its parts. This synergy creates opportunities for breakthroughs and development.

In a conversation, the generative potential could be the spark of insight or a new solution that arises when participants are engaged in a deep, open, and non-judgmental exchange. It's about what can emerge rather than what *already is*.

In attuning to the generative potential in Dialogue, the facilitator's emphasis is on allowing the unfolding of something new and vital, which can only happen when there's openness, trust, and a readiness to embrace uncertainty within the Dialogue. Navigating the unknown is an integral role of the facilitator, constantly differentiating between systems awareness, knowledge of methods and both a personal and relationship-focused practice. Facilitators need to embody personal qualities such as unconditional positive regard, empathic understanding and congruence, and to be able to be helpful at times of uncertainty and systemic complexity (von Korff, 2024).

THE AUTISM DIALOGUE APPROACH: TRAINING FOR FACILITATORS

The Autism Dialogue Approach (ADA) training course is based on training that our specialist autism trainers have been delivering successfully to hundreds of professionals across the UK and internationally for some years. The course offers a comprehensive understanding of autism and the ADA framework. This framework comprises principles that establish a structure for providing the best support. The training emphasises autistic perspectives and teaches how to tailor strategies to ensure optimal support and comprehension in your organisation or community. Our training has been developed by a team of mostly autistic people and is delivered by highly trained and experienced facilitators. Bridging the gap across different neurotypes takes a lot of effort, experience and skill.

After modules on autistic communication, sensory experiences, intersectionality, trauma and others, delegates will hear about the latest autism-led scientific research, and then learn experientially to integrate a set of dialogic practices into existing skills.

Dialogic pedagogy is designed on equity, meaning participants are equals while bringing their whole selves to training, integrating personal values while reflecting on real-world work-based examples. A more embodied knowing and increased confidence means they will find it easier to authentically reach people with different modes of being. This increases trust, improves communication and produces more vital relationships, thereby generating more insight and healing together.

QUALITIES OF AN ADA-TRAINED PRACTITIONER

- A high level of self-awareness.
- Always aware of power imbalances.
- Constantly neuro-affirming awareness and practice.
- Sensing into autism, trauma, and autistic trauma.
- Prioritise the needs and experiences while eschewing normative social expectations.
- Knowing and embodying the Four Practices of Dialogue.

The focus of the Autism Dialogue practitioner is a return towards the dialogical environment itself. We experience the world and are healed through relationships. Connection lies at the core of Dialogue. Authenticity and trust are requirements in any relationship, and we need to meet the people we support exactly where they are; to raise their voices as equals thereby reaching positive, collaborative outcomes together. This course is in constant development. At the time of writing, certification is not available, although this is being explored and might be by the time you're reading this.

AUTISTIC-ONLY GROUP?

Autistic-only dialogues are important for several reasons, but ADA is not a platform for strengthening sub-cultures. There are many of this kind of group already. ADA works on the principle of micro-macro – that of reflecting the wider community or society.

However, many, if not most autistic people need to own and see autism as part of their identity – which means identifying with other autistics. Some of the principles of Dialogue can certainly be used for this purpose.

South African Dialogue facilitator Helena Wagener clarified this to me when she suggested there might be a need to build an embodied resilience for difficult dialogues as well as dialogic skills that are more in line with autistic preferences – so that autistic participants feel empowered to come into dialogue with non-autistic counterparts (i.e. therapists/healthcare workers and other professionals).

Similarly, parallel training could happen to build resilience and dialogic skills in professionals to be present with autistic participants from a place that is less defensive or anxious, then only in the end would one bring the two groups together to dialogue (H. Wagener, personal correspondence, 23 September 2024)

If we consider the aim of a holistic society, where autistic people are integrated and included rather than excluded, then we can see how resilience dialogues would be important – as a stage on the way to holistic cohesion across society.

To support the all-inclusive group model, one autistic participant provided the following feedback: 'I didn't like that non autistic people were present. It didn't feel appropriate to share issues outside of an all autistic group' (personal correspondence, 2020).

WORKING WITH AN ORGANISATION

> It is actually quite rare for leaders in business to dedicate time to exploring their own thinking processes, and indeed, it is not easy for them to accept that this could ever be part of developing more effective business methods.
> *(Robinson, 2020, para. 11)*

Group dialogue processes can be time-consuming, which may not be ideal for fast-paced or urgent professional situations. Dialogues in organisations often involve extensive discussions and consensus-building, which can slow down decision-making processes.

Here's a suggestion for working with an organisation, which I loosely used several times.

1. Consult – client consultation.
2. Gather – interviews with key stakeholders.
3. Recruit/invite – recruitment/invitation event.
4. Generate – series of generative dialogues – including process (4-stage intergroup model).
5. Produce – co-production of report.

6. Present – final dialogue/presentation event.
7. Follow – follow-up consultation.

1. Consult – client consultation

Leaders of complex organisations come to us in many ways whereby both formal and informal conversations might continue for several weeks or even months before the chemistry between parties is right, the time is right for both, the benefits are understood (including by commissioners) and an invitation is put forward. Once the contract is agreed upon, a named representative at the organisation is selected who will be the point of contact between Dialogica and the prospective participants to be invited to a programme. It is important that their role in mediating between the cohort and Dialogica is sensitive and some pre-conversation in this regard might be necessary.

2. Gather – interviews

Short interviews with selected stakeholders, including leaders and clients, are held by the dialogue facilitators. They are semi-formal and usually guided by an open question generated by the client's initial consultation brief. These inform the facilitators with some information and current views about the prevailing system. Improved understanding and relations with individuals in the cohort prior to the group work allow for greater familiarity with the work and participants overall. Subtle characteristics of both individual and systemic influences are absorbed by the interviewers, who are then better equipped as facilitators.

3. Recruit – recruitment event

Presentation of the client's brief in the context of ADA to potential participants including leadership. Buy-in from all members of the organisation is crucial to capture a full picture, inform everyone and holistically address dynamics including inherent power.

Stages 2 and 3 may be swapped, depending on the situation.

4. Generate – a series of generative dialogues

This is the core of the programme and where the ADA is implemented (see above). It will usually consist of between six and 10, (two to three hours) sessions. Participants are guided by practices and principles via communication from the facilitators, as they prepare to enter the first session. The facilitators aim to be accepted as working with the group (rather than 'for' or 'to') and whose demonstration of the principles and trust are key to creating a safe and welcoming environment. Virtual and physical venues will be made familiar to all via electronic means. Standard informalities will be in place such as coffee and 'foyer-talk', but with heightened awareness and sensitivities of the typical anxieties created by such environments in neurodivergent people. The facilitators will be helping to create the required atmosphere conducive to the desired outcomes and aware that 'autism-friendly' means different things to different people. Facilitators are contactable directly by participants throughout the programme, but will not engage in any of the content brought to the confidential dialogues.

5. Produce – co-production of report

Facilitators write a draft report and go through a step-by-step process liaising with the cohort until a final report is agreed upon. The report will typically include a background, remit, aims and objectives, methods, timeline, anonymous quotes, themes (e.g. autism, the system, personal), outcomes and next steps with suggestions from the organisation.

6. Present – final dialogue/presentation event

The report will be put into slide form and a webinar presentation will be followed by a final Q&A style dialogue with the organisation's wider networks and stakeholders and if appropriate, the public.

7. Follow – follow up consultation

At a mutually agreed time, usually one month after the presentation event.

PROFESSIONAL DIALOGUE

There is no formal training or certification required to practise Autism Dialogue, and anyone can become an Autism Dialogue Professional, regardless of their background or qualifications. Dialogue goes beyond method; it is a natural, adaptive process that evolves based on the circumstances.

The efficacy and effectiveness of professional dialogue are becoming increasingly evident in addressing fundamental problems in many areas of society. The Academy of Professional Dialogue has demonstrated this in recent years with its events and publications to which I've contributed (Drury, 2019; Drury, Salinsky & Elliott, 2022). Dialogue encourages diverse individuals with different backgrounds, experiences, and viewpoints to come together and share their thoughts. This diversity can lead to innovative solutions and a deeper understanding of complex issues. Participating in dialogue can help people improve their communication skills, including active listening, empathy, and effective speaking. These skills are valuable in various professional settings. Group dialogue can provide a structured platform for constructively addressing conflicts and disagreements, promoting open and honest discussions that can lead to consensus or compromise. In professional contexts, group dialogue can aid in informed decision-making. It allows for the exploration of multiple options and the evaluation of potential consequences before reaching a conclusion. Engaging in group dialogue can foster a sense of community and teamwork among participants. This can lead to stronger professional relationships and collaboration.

Dialogue is open to everyone and enhances any setting where evolving and interactive experiences are underway. It can effortlessly blend into your life, indeed becoming a set of principles to live by, and many who begin using dialogue in their own work often develop a passion for sharing it with others. Autism Dialogue facilitation, and how it will be taught will not be standardised. Frozen structures are antithetical to the ethics of dialogue and it is a core value of Autism Dialogue that the diversity of approaches will be protected. Constructive critiques are welcome among our leadership or between practitioners, facilitators and individuals presenting or applying practices which arise from Bohm's philosophy of the implicit. These should be offered by means of open, respectful communication. Your organisation will seek to honour the value of diversity of approaches in its offerings.

If you want to become an Autism Dialogue Professional, begin by learning the basics. Once you're ready to go deeper, you'll perhaps want to attend a training course (see www.dialogica.uk).

REFERENCES

Benford, P. & Standen, P. (2009). The internet: a comfortable communication medium for people with Asperger syndrome (AS) and high functioning autism (HFA)? *Journal of Assistive Technologies*, 3(2), 44–53. https://doi.org/10.1108/17549450200900015

Carroll, M. (2011). Ethical maturity: compasses for life and work decisions-Part I. *Psychotherapy in Australia*, 17, 34.

Cuffari, E., Fourlas, G. N. & Whatley, M. (n.d.). Enactive ethics. Retrieved from www.elenaclarecuffari.com/research/enactive-ethics

Drury, J. (2019) Autism Dialogue. In C. Penwell (ed.), *The World Needs Dialogue! One: Gathering the Field* (pp. 293–304). Dialogue Publications.

Drury, J., Salinsky, K. & Elliott, J. (2022) Autism Dialogue in Derby City and Derbyshire. In H. Wagener & C. Penwell (eds), *The World Needs Dialogue! Four: Putting Dialogue to Work* (pp. 83–88). Dialogue Publications.

Foulkes, S. H., & Anthony, E. J. (2018). *Group Psychotherapy: The Psychoanalytic Approach* (2nd edition). Routledge.

Heider, J. (2015). *The Tao of Leadership: Lao Tzu's Tao Te Ching Adapted for a New Age*. Green Dragon Books.

National Autistic Society. (2017, March 28). Make it stop [video]. Retrieved from www.youtube.com/watch?v=xHHwZJX67-M

Newson, M., Zhao, Y., Zein, M.E., Sulik, J., Dezecache, G., Deroy, O. & Tunçgenç, B. (2021). Digital contact does not promote wellbeing, but face-to-face contact does: a cross-national survey during the COVID-19 pandemic. *New Media and Society*, 26(1). https://doi.org/10.1177/14614448211062164

Robinson, S. (2020). The inspiration of infinite potential: the life and ideas of David Bohm. Retrieved from https://transitionconsciousness.wordpress.com/2020/06/21/the-inspiration-of-infinite-potential-the-life-and-ideas-of-david-bohm/

von Korff, Y. (2024). *A Practical Guide to Group Facilitation: The Threefold Approach*. Routledge.

Wijers, L. (ed.) (1996). *Art Meets Science and Spirituality in a Changing Economy: From Competition to Compassion*. Academy Editions.

PART III

Wider contexts

CHAPTER 12

Intersectionality and Dialogue

....

In this chapter, I describe the concept of intersectionality and its complex relationship to autism and neurodiversity and provide some background to Intergroup Dialogue (IGD). In closing, I've provided some background into recent work combining the above and offered some thoughts about how IGD and the Autism Dialogue Approach (ADA) compare.

In the same way as this book is intended to activate and support Dialogues about autism, this chapter could provide a starting point for dialogues about autism and intersectionality.

Intersectionality is a framework first introduced by black legal scholar Kimberlé Crenshaw in the late 1980s. It recognises how various aspects of a person's identity, including race, gender, sexuality, disability and more, intersect and influence their experiences of privilege and oppression. Crenshaw (1989) says the point of intersectionality is to make room for more advocacy and remedial practices to create a more egalitarian system. Thinking about intersectionality can help in understanding autistic people's different experiences, especially in terms of how their experiences are influenced by different aspects of society. Here's a great example of both positive and negative impacts of intersectionality:

> I love being an autistic, Muslim Pakistani woman. My identity in itself is so diverse, which I am really proud of! It does make it harder to live so freely however, with all of the stigma and discrimination that surrounds both autistic people and Muslims. Race and autism intersect a lot and talking about race in autism conversations is so important.
>
> (Iqra Babar, cited in National Autistic Society, n.d., para. 13)

There has been some constructive criticism of the intersectionality model, as well as simple misunderstandings, embedded in the assumption that someone's claims of discrimination or exclusion are unidirectional. However, intersectionality simply means someone can experience discrimination in multiple ways, as Crenshaw explains with the analogy of an intersection or crossroads:

> Consider an analogy to traffic in an intersection, coming and going in all four directions. Discrimination, like traffic through an intersection, may flow in one direction, and it may flow in another. If an accident happens in an intersection, it can be caused by cars traveling from any number of directions and, sometimes, from all of them. Similarly, if a Black woman is harmed because she is in the intersection, her injury could result from sex discrimination or race discrimination.
>
> *(Crenshaw, 1989, p. 149)*

Autistic people who belong to additional marginalised groups, whether through race, ethnicity, gender identity, sexual orientation, or disability can face multiple layers of discrimination and exclusion. The intersection of these identities shapes their experiences in ways that create unique and complex challenges and for many; the realities of being different are compounded by the fact that their differences are often invisible to others, while some such as skin colour or certain disability are hypervisible. This invisibility can result in misunderstandings, stigma and the erasure of their identity, leaving their specific needs unmet.

The barriers faced are often made worse by limited access to healthcare, education, employment, and essential support services. The disparities are not just about being autistic or neurodivergent – they're intensified by other intersecting aspects of identity, deepening the inequalities they encounter.

Cultural and contextual factors also play a significant role. Depending on societal expectations and norms, the experience of being autistic can vary widely. Intersectionality helps us to understand how these cultural dimensions influence how individuals are perceived and treated, and how their needs can be overlooked within their communities.

In a form of medicalised racism just a few hundred years ago, enslaved people who attempted to escape were often labelled with 'drapetomania' for daring to flee their enslavers (Eltis et al., 2017). This fabricated mental illness category was used as propaganda to uphold the social order, driven by the fears of the ruling classes and slave owners.

The environment and dominant social values remain influenced by deeply ingrained narratives of what is perceived as illness. A person with multiple marginalised identities can be treated with violence instead of care, respect and consideration of their autonomy and rights. Binary thinking involves categorising people as 'abled' or 'disabled' and placing ourselves as 'the helper' versus 'the helped'. These binaries are pervasive and shape who accesses support and care, and many people whom society claims to care for already come with a reputation attached. It is fairly common for a word like 'aggressive' to be used in a report carelessly, by just one staff member who describes a single incident when they witnessed a distressed patient.

Dialogue is a powerful tool to examine and expand how we tell these stories, and how we place ourselves within the stories of others. Through Dialogue, we can disrupt harmful narratives and create meaningful connections.

Intersectionality is crucial in bringing to light the nuanced, layered experiences of many people. It is focused on social justice and like the Autism Dialogue Approach, aims to equalise power in all areas of society and level the societal playing field. 'Intersectionality operates as both the observance and analysis of power imbalances and the tool by which those power imbalances could be eliminated altogether'. (Coaston, 2019, para. 48).

To address the oppression faced by autistic people with intersecting minority identities, we may approach the issue from multiple angles while remembering the dialogic notion that *right action follows right thinking*, and not the other way round. 'Within critical autism studies, a field that emerged to challenge the deficit-laden, pathologizing autism discourses favored by the medical community, intersectionality has started to become an integral component of the literature' (Mallipeddi & VanDaalen, 2022, p. 281).

Dialogue facilitators must be highly aware of their own privileges and disadvantages in order to genuinely empathise with a wide and dynamic range of people and their intersecting identities. Spaces must be inclusive and accessible, ensuring the ability to share concerns without fear of exclusion or dismissal. Advocacy is key to Dialogue so the facilitator's self-awareness and moral conscience need to be well refined. A useful concept for facilitator's to be aware of is multi-partiality, which involves holding multiple stories and perspectives while recognising that all the needs within a group are important. In terms of Dialogue facilitation, this is described as being on everyone's side.

Support organisations should recognise the distinct challenges faced and create environments where all voices are truly heard. Raising awareness in words and actions can help dismantle stigma and foster greater understanding and when carried out with sensitivity and genuineness, can be highly effective. Workshops, training programs, and public campaigns can bring issues into focus, helping to create a more compassionate, informed programme, therefore society, and up-to-date social awareness are paramount for organisers of Dialogues.

Inclusive policies are essential in breaking down systemic barriers. Whether in education, healthcare, or employment, policies that promote diversity, equity, and inclusion must be designed with input from the very individuals they aim to support. Without their voices, these efforts risk missing the mark. Cultural competence and understanding the unique cultural and intersectional needs of autistic people ensures they receive the support they require in ways that respect and honour their identities.

INTERGROUP DIALOGUE

Intergroup Dialogue (IGD) began at the University of Michigan in the 1980s as a way to bring diverse groups of students, faculty, and staff together to address racial tensions on campus. IGD is a facilitated person-to-person learning experience that brings together individuals from different social identity groups to explore similarities and differences. Its goal is to examine social inequalities and foster collaboration across diverse perspectives. Co-facilitation, often by individuals with distinct identities, mirrors the approach of Autism Dialogue (ADA), which requires at least one autistic facilitator. This method promotes safety, and diverse representation, and models how to navigate systemic tensions. As the dialogue progresses, participants take a more active role, with facilitators stepping back to encourage a more decentralised and collaborative process.

IGD is a research-based model that blends theory and practice, using knowledge of social identities, oppression, and justice to promote social change. It works on the premise that constructive processing of conflict can lead to the learning and empowerment of marginalised groups.

Because IGD comes from the United States with its unique race dynamic, this is one of the main underpinnings of the practice. However, IGD has been used extensively between persons and groups of different genders, religions, abilities, socioeconomic classes etc. Many universities and community groups in the USA use IGD. According to the University of Michigan, IGD facilitators should be trained in expert listening skills and in empathy skills, have been well trained in advance in the specific techniques of dialogue, be experienced in ongoing processes of exploring their own attitudes and behaviours regarding diversity and justice and should know how to share power and create democratic, non-authoritarian environments (Gurin, Nagada & Zúñiga, 2013).

IGD is structured in four stages and is designed to build trust and group cohesion over time. It allows participants to gradually engage in more challenging conversations as the group becomes more comfortable with each other. The goal is to transform differences, not by eliminating them, but by drawing them in to form stronger social relationships – a crucial process for promoting critical thinking and social justice.

Focussing on intergroup dialogue pedagogy developed by the University of Michigan, a three-year multi-university field experiment was undertaken, examining the effects of intergroup dialogue pedagogy at nine universities. Evidence shows that contact between groups can lead to decreased prejudice and stereotyping if conditions of 'good contact' are met, which include superordinate goals, alternatives to normative roles and power distributions, sustained interaction that embraces issues of group difference, etc. (Gurin et al., 2013).

One key point in IGD is that individuals are encouraged to avoid speaking for an entire group or advocating or educating others on behalf of that group. That's a lot of pressure when someone is the only one representing an identity group, especially for black participants, given the specific historical context. Practitioners strive not to have just one person from any racial or ethnic group in a session. IGD draws heavily from the US Civil Rights Movement and thinkers of all colours as well as individual identities, and is also about power, oppression, and how different identities hold power within social hierarchies. The way these dynamics blend and play out in various systems of power is a crucial focus of IGD.

The four stages of IGD usually take place over 12–16 weeks but can be adapted to different timeframes, including one-off sessions. The first stage involves introductions, creating group guidelines and reflecting on and sharing social identities. This builds community. In the second stage intersectionality is explored. In the third stage, participants discuss 'hot topics', which are often difficult, controversial issues brought up by the group. Finally, in the fourth stage, there is a focus on action, encouraging participants to apply what they've learned through individual or collective action projects (UHRI, 2017).

THE CYCLES OF SOCIALISATION AND LIBERATION

The 'Cycle of Socialisation' and the 'Cycle of Liberation' (Harro, 2000) are two conceptual frameworks common to Intergroup Dialogue. These provide insight into one's own socialising (where one is usually 'acting from a place of fear or scarcity') towards liberation and the final goal of acting from a place of radical love and applying 'right action' within the self and one's relationships to co-create systems that work for more people. Harro's model speaks to the different approaches participants can take, starting with personal work. Dialogue helps sustain the journey, offering a grounding practice of checking in with a group and moving away from individualism.

> **My experience in Intergroup Dialogue**
>
> Understanding neurodiversity and intersectionality together in a way that promotes inclusion, reflection and action requires a framework to explore these complexities, bringing our stories and identities into conversation with others and creating new pathways for understanding. As an IGD course participant, I became deeply aware of my own sensitivity and realised that different people experience varying levels of sensitivity and that this shapes how they engage with concepts like bravery and curiosity; therefore these words started losing their definition for me, which felt rather unsettling. This experience led me to reach out to the training organisation and we formulated a programme to address this aspect, bringing autism and neurodiversity into the IGD sphere.

IGD emphasises equitable participation and participants strive for mutual comprehension of diverse viewpoints in a non-judgmental atmosphere. By examining preconceptions and biases within peer groups and focusing on group division and socialisation, it aims to potentially lead to insights and deeper understanding among individuals within those groups. While aspects of IGD would be useful in the social context for uniting autistic and non-autistic groupings, Bohm Dialogue has more focus on fragmentation of consciousness and thought and therefore has a stronger alignment with autism and the nature of the self, which includes the context of social groups.

In this age of communication-meta-crisis and fragmentation of consciousness, struggles for identity assertion reach fever pitch. We are charged with difficult and complex questions of change, forcing us to examine and reveal deeply held, often unconscious beliefs, even about our identity groupings. In elevating and encouraging dialogue among peers to speak openly and honestly, modelling disagreements around isms, intersections and potential conflicts among them, it seems to me that we also need to go within, to the nature of self, in an equal measure, Bohm's (1980) theory of Implicate Order and his evolving Dialogue modalities allows us to do just that. Combinations of both personal and impersonal, inner and outer dimensions of communication in an integration of Bohm/Autism Dialogue Approach and Intergroup Dialogue would be useful to explore further.

Intergroup Dialogue allows the complexity of intersectional identities to enfold and unfold naturally. The Autism Dialogue Approach redefines inclusion by focusing on the whole person, demonstrating that true inclusion not only makes room for different perspectives but is about creating spaces where deep personal insight and change is facilitated and resulting perspectives can immediately (and meaningfully) influence the group.

Exercise: questions to ponder

- What do autism, race, power and similar concepts mean to you, as a person and/or a professional?
- How do these play out and influence your work, practice and your life?
- What are your own stories of inner and outer transformation?
- What unknown influences might you be bringing to your relationships at work and personal life?
- Where can we find the answers?

As you reflect on these questions, ask, what can you do to remain steadfast to yourself as an agent of change, and as part of a whole, dynamic process?

REFERENCES

Bohm, D. (1980). *Wholeness and the Implicate Order.* Routledge & Kegan Paul.
Coaston, J. (2019). The intersectionality wars. Retrieved from www.vox.com/the-highlight/2019/5/20/18542843/intersectionality-conservatism-law-race-gender-discrimination
Crenshaw, K. (1989). Demarginalizing the intersection of race and sex: a black feminist critique of antidiscrimination doctrine. *University of Chicago Legal Forum*, 1989(1), article 8.
Eltis, D., Engerman, S. L., Drescher, S. & Richardson, D. (eds). (2017). *Slavery. In The Cambridge World History of Slavery* (pp. 71–318). Cambridge: Cambridge University Press.
Gurin, P., Nagda, B. (R.) A. & Zúñiga, X. (2013). *Dialogue across Difference: Practice, Theory, and Research on Intergroup Dialogue.* Russell Sage Foundation.
Harro, B. (2000). The Cycle of Liberation. In M. Adams, W. Blumenfeld, R. Casteñeda, H. Hackman, M. L. Peters, & X. Zuniga (eds), *Readings for Diversity and Social Justice* (p. 464). Routledge.

Mallipeddi, N. V. & VanDaalen, R. A. (2022). Intersectionality within critical autism studies: a narrative review. *Autism in Adulthood*, 4(4), 281–289. https://doi.org/10.1089/aut.2021.0014

National Autistic Society. (n.d.). Stories from the spectrum: Iqra Babar. Retrieved from www.autism.org.uk/advice-and-guidance/stories/stories-from-the-spectrum-iqra-babar

UHRI. (2017). Facilitated Intergroup Dialogue. Retrieved from www.uhri.ngo/facilitated-intergroup-dialogue

CHAPTER 13

Insight Dialogue and other models

....

We've looked at autism's atypical way of being, as well as the predominant deficit perspective and theories like the double empathy problem, which attempts to explain the tensions of relating to another neuro-type. Everyone has in common the limitations of using language, which, as well as being culture-bound and (in English at least) rather noun-based, is constantly influenced by fractured systems, resulting in fragmented thought, agendas, lies, warped ideologies, cross-purposes, values-clashes and other barriers to understanding. We don't have to look far to appreciate the amount of confusion implicit in modern communication.

The question that's sometimes asked of the practice of Autism Dialogue is about the notion of continuing impact in one's life, out in the community and in society. As Dialogues are closed groups based on agreement among peers, communication with others who are not practitioners, or those who are unaware of the practice of Dialogue, has implications. However, going out about our daily business and meeting people like shopkeepers, teachers, neighbours and so on doesn't require deep levels of awareness as we exchange communication for what is needed from each other. But the practice of Dialogue affects our being and this, in turn, affects others and our relationships. Embodying the 'four practices' of dialogue (authentic voice, deep listening, respecting and suspending) can be a good way to live while relating with the world at large.

On the topic of awareness, if we agree that the aim of what we call mindfulness is to return us to our own natural aware state, the purpose of a meditation practice is to increase and cultivate that awareness into our lives, with the aim of increasing natural empowerment and satisfaction.

Taking this into our relationships, Insight Dialogue founder Gregory Kramer suggests that being in actual relational contact with another is mostly considered 'too challenging to recall our awareness, and beyond the domain of meditative practice'(Kramer, 2007). Kramer draws from Vipassana ('insight') Meditation and

Insight Dialogue invites us to consider if it's possible to not only recall, but cultivate presence in the moments of contact with another person.

Participants practise mindfulness in conversation, with an emphasis on staying present, aware, and responsive to others in a reflective, kind, and non-reactive manner. Kramer sought to bring the insights gained in silent meditation into the context of relational communication. The practice is rooted in Theravada Buddhism, particularly in the Brahma Viharas (the 'Divine Abodes') – qualities like compassion, loving-kindness, empathetic joy, and equanimity – which are essential in fostering mindful dialogue.

Insight Dialogue evolved to emphasise a set of key instructions: pause, relax, open, trust emergence, listen deeply, and speak the truth. These guidelines help individuals maintain awareness and presence while communicating, enhancing interpersonal understanding and emotional resilience. The Autism Dialogue Approach and Insight Dialogue are compared in Table 13.1.

TABLE 13.1 Comparison of Autism Dialogue and Insight Dialogue.

Autism Dialogue	Insight Dialogue
• 'Four practices': respect/suspend/listen/authentic voice and (added in 2019): 'slow the pace, make some space'. • Encourages participants to deeply listen and be present, cultivating a non-judgmental space for authentic expression. • Aims to create an environment where neurodivergent individuals feel heard and understood by others and promote relational understanding. • Values the co-creation of a safe, inclusive environment, where participants are encouraged to speak without fear of judgement and lean into compassion and embracing differences. • Slows down the pace of conversation to allow for careful reflection and to accommodate different communication styles. • Explore topics related to autism and neurodiversity collectively, learning from each other's lived experiences in an open-ended, emergent way.	• 'Six instructions': pause/relax/open/trust emergence/listen deeply/speak the truth. • Cultivates deep interpersonal connections through structured mindfulness in conversations. • Relationships between dialogue partners are central, as they co-create a space of trust and understanding. • Encourages participants to suspend judgement and meet others with compassion and acceptance, aligning with Buddhist principles of non-attachment and loving-kindness. • Promotes pauses and reflective silence, allowing participants to mindfully consider their words and the impact of their communication, fostering deep listening and thoughtful responses. • Aims to cultivate shared wisdom by engaging in conversations that allow mutual learning and insight, often centred on mindful awareness and the human experience.

Aspects in this table unique to Autism Dialogue are the slowing down of the conversational pace (added by participants in a 2019 programme) compared to 'pause' and 'reflective silence' in Insight Dialogue) and the suggestion of actually exploring autism and neurodiversity. Both approaches have a strong implicit focus on slowing down thought and communication processes to enhance mutual respect and deeper understanding, allowing participants to connect across differences and explore their shared humanity to cultivate mutual growth. 'Slowing down' is made explicit in Autism Dialogue, recognising the impact of a fast-paced world upon autistic and highly sensitive people. 'Respect' is also an unmentioned 'given' in Insight Dialogue, which deserves some consideration in terms of what respect for the other really is. It seems that the subtle differences which appear in Autism Dialogue relate to what autistic people need (slower communication and better respect), and recovery, rather than the desires of the general population wishing to increase awareness and improve awareness in relationships *per se*.

Mindful communication approaches like Insight Dialogue can improve emotional regulation, reduce anxiety, and foster empathy, making it valuable for personal relationships, workplaces, and therapeutic settings. Neuroscientific research also supports the idea that mindfulness practices activate brain areas linked to empathy and self-awareness, which are crucial in social interaction and conflict resolution (see Chapter 9).

When considering the application of mindful dialogue for autism, the benefits are pronounced. Insight Dialogue offers a structured, mindful approach that addresses difficulties such as social interaction, communication, self-awareness and emotional regulation. By slowing the pace of communication and creating space for reflective, compassionate dialogue, Insight Dialogue can reduce sensory overwhelm and social anxiety. The practice promotes non-judgmental listening and acceptance, providing a safe and supportive environment where neurodiverse individuals feel heard and understood.

For society at large, Insight Dialogue's emphasis on connection and empathy makes it a powerful tool for integrating into Autism Dialogue, which aims to foster understanding across differences, specifically neurotypes. A continued use of a combined ADA-ID (ADA and Inter-Group Dialogue) approach in therapeutic and community settings could help bridge social divides, promote inclusivity, and support mental health, making it highly relevant in today's increasingly complex social landscape.

PEDAGOGY OF THE OPPRESSED

Also important in the combination of social domains and holistic awareness, one of the most influential works on Dialogue comes from Brazilian educator and philosopher Paulo Freire, particularly in his seminal book *Pedagogy of the Oppressed* (1970).

Freire introduced dialogue as a tool for fostering critical consciousness (*conscientização*). Through dialogue, individuals come to understand the social, political and economic contradictions in their reality. Rather than passively accepting information, participants in dialogue engage in critical thinking and reflection. This is important for empowering people to challenge oppressive systems and encouraging active participation in their transformation. Freire posits that dialogue is essential for humanisation. In oppressive systems, both the oppressed and the oppressors are dehumanised. Dialogue as praxis allows individuals to work together to regain their humanity through collaboration and respect for each other's dignity. It is through dialogue that people engage in a co-creation of knowledge, seeing each other as equals in a shared learning experience.

In education, Freire's dialogue is central to the problem-posing method, as opposed to the banking model where students are passive recipients of knowledge. Through dialogue, students and teachers engage in a process of reflection, questioning and action. This transforms education from being a mere transfer of information to an active, participatory process of critical thinking and empowerment. In Freire's terms, praxis is reflection and action directed at the structures to be transformed.

Dialogue as praxis plays a critical role in social movements and activism, bringing individuals together to discuss their shared experiences of oppression and build collective strategies for change. This collaborative approach helps avoid 'top-down' models of leadership, making social change more sustainable and inclusive as all participants have a voice in shaping the movement.

Dialogue carries an ethical dimension, demanding that participants engage with each other in good faith, with respect, openness, and a willingness to listen, which is essential for building trust and achieving authentic communication. As an ethical praxis, dialogue fosters solidarity and a commitment to the common good, rather than self-interest.

For Freire, dialogue is the foundation of any liberatory practice – it is both the means and the method through which oppressed individuals and communities can reclaim their agency and create a more just world. Dialogue is a powerful tool for personal growth, social transformation, and education. It moves beyond mere talk to become an act of engagement that fosters critical thinking, mutual humanisation, and collective action.

DIALOGISM AND ETHICAL AND SPIRITUAL INTERACTION: BOHM, BUBER AND BAKHTIN

There are countless dialogue methods available, each offering unique ways to foster meaningful conversation, reflection, and inquiry. Some approaches, like the Socratic Seminar and World Café, share similarities in their focus on collaborative exploration and shared learning, while others, such as Insight Dialogue or Bohm Dialogue, dive deeper into the personal and contemplative dimensions of communication. Each method can be adapted to different contexts, depending on the goals and dynamics of the group. Non-Violent Communication (NVC) (Rosenberg, 2015) provides a suitable lead-in to spirituality in Autism Dialogue in Chapter 15.

As we explore and apply these diverse methods, it's clear that dialogue is not a one-size-fits-all practice; it requires mindful adaptation to meet the needs of the participants and the depth of the topics at hand.

In the realm of autism enquiry, some methods resonate more strongly. The depth at which some autistic people think is profound and often marked by a nuanced, detail-oriented, and highly reflective approach to understanding the world. This depth of thought can sometimes feel constrained by more conventional dialogue methods, which tend to favour quick exchanges or surface-level conversations in a world dominated by neuro-normative standards. For those who process information in a more deliberate and contemplative manner, Bohm Dialogue offers a fitting alternative (Bohm, 1996).

Bohm Dialogue is particularly useful in this context because it emphasises slowing down the conversation, allowing for deep reflection and careful articulation of ideas.

Its emphasis on suspending assumptions and listening deeply without judgement aligns with the need for spaces that honour neurodivergent communication styles. Its unstructured, flowing nature allows for the kind of slow, reflective engagement that can be particularly valuable in discussions around neurodiversity, where creating a sense of openness and understanding is crucial.

Its structure creates a space where complex, layered thinking can unfold without the pressure to reach immediate conclusions. This method nurtures the kind of open, patient inquiry that honours the way many autistic people engage with ideas – offering the time and space needed to explore thoughts with precision and depth. In a world that often prioritises speed and efficiency in communication, as well as activism and social engagement, Bohm Dialogue serves as a crucial reminder that true understanding often requires slowing down and giving each voice the space it needs to fully express its inner workings.

While Bohm focuses on dialogue as a means of collective inquiry to address societal fragmentation and foster shared meaning, there are significant contributions to Dialogue from Mikhail Bakhtin and Martin Buber. Each approached dialogue from a different perspective, but both shared a belief in its transformative and ethical importance and offered a unique lens on dialogue, reinforcing its importance as praxis for human development, understanding and ethical interaction.

Mikhail Bakhtin (1895–1975), a Russian philosopher and literary theorist, introduced the concept of dialogism. He argued that all language is inherently dialogic, meaning it involves a relationship between voices, each with its perspective and worldview. In a dialogic exchange, these multiple voices can engage in a dynamic interaction. Bakhtin's work highlights the importance of heteroglossia, or the presence of multiple voices and perspectives within discourse, which creates a richer, more nuanced understanding of meaning. This polyphonic view recognises that understanding is always co-created through interaction and tension between different perspectives (Bakhtin, 1981). Bakhtin posited that Dialogue is fundamental to meaning-making and the construction of identity, as it involves the interaction of multiple, sometimes conflicting, voices.

Martin Buber (1878–1965), a Jewish philosopher, is famous for his distinction between 'I–thou' and 'I–it' relationships. In an 'I–thou' relationship, individuals engage with each other as whole, unique beings, while in an 'I–it' relationship, the other is seen as an object to be used or analysed. Dialogue, for Buber, is the core of the 'I–thou' relationship, where participants encounter each other authentically and fully. This type of dialogue fosters genuine connection and mutual recognition of the other's humanity. It is not instrumental, but ethical and spiritual, aiming to create real contact between persons (Buber, 1937).

CIRCLES OF TRUST

The Circles of Trust concept is influenced by the Quaker 'Clearness Committee' (Quakers, 2012) and is grounded in the work of educator and writer Parker J. Palmer, particularly as outlined in his book *A Hidden Wholeness: The Journey Toward an Undivided Life* (2004).

Circles are intended to be safe spaces where people can explore their inner truths, engage in deep reflection and foster authentic dialogue with others. They are for one individual to discern a difficult life decision or inner conflict where a group asks open-ended questions but avoids offering advice or direction, trusting that the individual has the inner resources to find clarity. Questions are considered more important than answers and are intended to help the person clarify their own thinking rather than leading them to a specific conclusion.

The key principles draw on a mixture of Quaker traditions, principles of communal discernment, and non-coercive facilitation. Silence, reflection and the inner teacher are central elements and the process emphasises non-hierarchical forms of discernment, where every individual's experience and inner wisdom are valued equally. This echoes principles of 'communal discernment' often found in spiritual traditions.

Palmer emphasises deep listening and respect for individual journeys. The goal is not to offer solutions or advice but to hold space for people to reflect on their inner lives and experiences (Palmer, 2004). Participants are encouraged to use periods of silence to listen to their inner voice, what Palmer calls the inner teacher. This practice draws from the Quaker tradition of silent worship, where moments of quiet contemplation are central to discernment and deep spiritual reflection.

Dialogue in Circles of Trust avoids debate or argument, fostering a 'third way' of engagement. This means that participants are not trying to persuade or convince, but are engaging in a form of dialogue without an agenda, which encourages open, honest exchanges without defensiveness.

Individuals 'hold tensions' and conflicting emotions gently, without trying to force resolution, allowing deeper understanding to emerge over time.

THE SOCRATIC SEMINAR

The Socratic Seminar is a structured group dialogue method rooted in the teaching philosophy of Socrates, the classical Greek philosopher who believed in the power of questioning to stimulate critical thinking and uncover underlying assumptions. In a Socratic Seminar, participants engage in a facilitated discussion centred around a shared text, question, or theme. Rather than aiming for definitive answers, the focus is on exploring ideas, asking probing questions, and deepening understanding through dialogue.

The term Socratic Seminar was first popularised by philosopher and educator Mortimer J. Adler in the mid-twentieth century. In his book, *The Paideia Proposal: An Educational Manifesto* (1982), he advocated for the Socratic Seminar as a central teaching method to foster critical thinking, intellectual development, and a love for inquiry. While Socratic questioning dates back to ancient Greece, it was Adler who formalised and coined the term Socratic Seminar as an educational practice. Adler's work built on Socratic principles, adapting them into a structured form of group dialogue where participants engage in questioning and collaborative inquiry, making it a widely adopted method in modern educational systems. As a dialogue method, it is particularly effective for exploring moral, ethical, or philosophical topics, but it can be adapted for a wide range of subjects. It creates an environment where participants feel empowered to question, challenge, and explore ideas in a supportive, thoughtful manner.

WORLD CAFÉ

The World Café draws on the metaphor of a café as a relaxed, open space for dialogue. It is designed to foster collaborative conversations around important questions, using small groups to encourage active participation and cross-pollination of ideas. Participants rotate between tables, discussing a common theme, and contribute to the collective exploration of ideas, which promotes collaboration, creative thinking and the emergence of new ideas through casual yet focused dialogue.

World Café originated in 1995, co-created by Juanita Brown and David Isaacs during a conversation among a group of colleagues at their home. Brown and Isaacs developed a more formalised set of principles and processes, which were published in their 2005 book *The World Café: Shaping Our Futures Through Conversations That Matter*.

REFERENCES

Adler, M. J. (1982). *The Paideia Proposal: An Educational Manifesto*. Macmillan.
Bakhtin, M. M. (1981). *The Dialogic Imagination: Four Essays*. University of Texas Press.
Bohm, D. (1996). *On Dialogue*. Routledge.
Brown, J. & Isaacs, D. (2005). *The World Café: Shaping Our Futures Through Conversations That Matter*. Berrett-Koehler Publishers.
Buber, M. (1937). *I and Thou* (2nd edition). Trans. R. G. Smith. Edinburgh: T. & T. Clark.
Freire, P. (1970). *Pedagogy of the Oppressed*. Seabury Press.
Kramer, G. (2007). *Insight Dialogue: The Interpersonal Path to Freedom*. Shambhala.
Palmer, P. J. (2004). *A Hidden Wholeness: The Journey Toward an Undivided Life*. Jossey-Bass.
Quakers. (2012). Clearness meeting guidance. Retrieved from www.quaker.org.uk/documents/clearness-meeting-guidance-2012.pdf
Rosenberg, M. B. (2015). *Nonviolent Communication: A Language of Life*. (3rd edition). PuddleDancer Press.

CHAPTER 14

Autism Dialogue in therapy and coaching

....

Therapy and coaching are very different but for this chapter, they come together and I frame them both within a Dialogic approach. In unfolding their commonalities, I offer suggestions for supporting autistic and neurodivergent individuals in the general professional helping spaces.

While commonly aimed at personal development, therapy, counselling and coaching serve distinct roles. Therapy focuses on healing and resolving past issues, typically to address mental health concerns, trauma, or emotional distress and will guide clients through psychological healing, helping them manage conditions such as anxiety, depression, or PTSD. Therapy may delve deep into a person's past, exploring how early experiences influence present behaviours.

Coaching, on the other hand, is largely future-focused. Coaches work with people to set and achieve specific goals, whether in personal growth, career development, or life transitions. While coaching can acknowledge the past, it doesn't dwell on it but uses it as a foundation for explicitly moving forward. The relationship in coaching is typically more collaborative, with clients considered the experts in their own lives. Gestalt coaching goes further and aligns with our autism-strengths-focused approach:

> The client is regarded from the start to be functioning as a whole, healthy, and resourceful entity with respect to environmental conditions. This attitude differentiates the activity of coaching from that of 'therapy,' which traditionally construes the client to be in some manner deficient and in need of regulated remediation.
>
> *(Siminovitch, & Van Eron, n.d., para. 7)*

The key difference lies in the purpose: therapy often addresses dysfunction to restore emotional wellbeing, while coaching focuses on unlocking potential and creating actionable plans. Coaching is not a substitute for therapy but can complement it for individuals looking to thrive after working through deeper emotional challenges. But all of these definitions reflect normalcy and autism is not the normality we are exploring, especially in anything which relates to 'Autism Dialogue'.

AUTISM AND EXISTENCE

As in life, autistic people in therapy or coaching struggle with a key problem: how and when do I be 'me'? And in these settings the question can be enhanced.

All of the known helping approaches can be transformative and all are essentially dialogic. In taking a social constructionist perspective, Armstrong (2012, p. 33) proposes that 'dialogue is the flow of meaning between human beings as they interact' and they are the meaning-makers of their own situation. This aligns with the enactivist perspective of humans as 'linguistic bodies' which assumes a deep continuity between life and mind and language, that each of us is a linguistic body in a community of other linguistic bodies.

Something I've discovered through experience that 'the difference between therapy and coaching is overstated' (Bader, 2009, para. 1). In fact, many if not most autistic people who attend coaching with me usually reveal the need for recovery first and tend to veer towards the existential – beyond standardised categories of therapy and coaching.

> Is society healthy, that an individual should return to it? Has not society itself helped to make the individual unhealthy? Of course, the unhealthy must be made healthy, that goes without saying; but why should the individual adjust himself to an unhealthy society? If he is healthy, he will not be a part of it. Without first questioning the health of society, what is the good of helping misfits to conform to society?
>
> *(Krishnamurti, 1960, cited by Krishnamurti Foundation, n.d.)*

Recently there's been a significant shift in our cultural demographics; this has exposed diversity needs, bringing waves of diversity awareness training. Professional helpers struggle to address the needs of a new generation of equity-deserving client groups.

Power in the therapy space remains with the therapist, due largely to assumed authority and unconscious bias. In hidden disabilities, for example, an attitude of 'different not deficient' is becoming popular, but looking behind the language of well-meaning, 'different' usually means from a white, western position and therefore embraces 'othering', for which long-term mental health implications are profoundly serious. I addressed this in Chapter 12 on Intersectionality. There appears to be a misuse of predominantly normative modes of therapy for autistic and neurodivergent populations.

Many helping professionals face major challenges when interacting across the neurotype divide, possibly even re-traumatising their autistic clients and patients.

This is largely to do with the inclination to adapt the protocol to account for autism and neurodiversity as a collection of deficits and, despite widespread concerns and protestations around the double empathy problem (Milton, 2012), the 'lacking a theory of mind' myth persists.

TALKING

On the whole, health care professionals, including psychologists, psychotherapists, counsellors and occupational and speech therapists, mostly emphasise verbal communication hence the term 'talking therapies'. Also, many therapies were researched and designed for individuals with a 'normal' brain, with assumptions about language. But what is normal communication, when we consider the impact of our environments, particularly upon autistic people? This is a difficult question that helpers must ask themselves as part of ethical consciousness and professional development. Let's take a brief look at what's happening in therapy. Many health professionals including therapists have attended our training programmes and revealed a surprising and unfortunate picture, where most have received little or no basic training in autism, or even neurodiversity awareness.

We take language and talking for granted, both in our dominant world cultures and in everyday spaces. When working with autistic people, respect and validation of different ways of perceiving and communicating is crucial, but how is it done?

Some practical ideas:

- Slowing down.
- Appreciating silence together, providing time to focus on topics of high interest (and leaning into them).
- Think about engaging other senses; many people, especially children, often communicate nonverbally through play, touch, and presence. Verbal or written communication is highly valued but in autistic culture not so much. Maintaining high levels of relational attuning, however, isn't done with any helper's toolkit.

AN ENACTIVE APPROACH TO THE HELPING RELATIONSHIP

Based on trust and personal bonds, the therapeutic relationship is considered to be the most significant factor in achieving positive therapeutic change (Paul & Charura, 2015) with the evolving relational model allowing clients to reshape their past and form healthier relationships in the present.

An attuned therapist or coach, with genuine curiosity, offers new perspectives not only on the self but also on the relationship, creating a safe space for the client to explore their story and form what Dr Daniel Siegel (2011) calls a 'coherent narrative'.

This process fosters secure attachments and trust. However, when autism is seen as a socially constructed idea of difference, we ought to reconsider what defines a trusting therapeutic relationship. What if the therapist's training lacked any meaningful understanding of autism, or what if the therapist and client are neurologically very different according to neurodiversity, with fundamentally contrasting worldviews? Autism, the nature of self, intersectionality and the neurodiversity paradigm are all now 'in the room', which can be deeply unsettling, resulting in reliance on toolkits and unconscious usage of systemic power.

Enactive theory, particularly its emphasis on participatory sense-making, offers a profound reimagining of therapeutic relationships. Traditional models, such as humanistic or person-centred therapies mostly do not take into account nuances of autism culture, unwritten rules and expectations of society and the therapy context for the 'client' or 'patient', and impacts of social expectations (being a good client or even self-justifying payment by referring to an internalised stereotype). Most therapists I've asked have little to no training in autism and its communication differences and sensory and social sensitivities. Alexithymia (difficulty understanding one's emotions) (Kinnaird et al., 2019; Kiraz et al., 2021) and rejection sensitive disorder (RSD) (Ginapp et al., 2023) are two common co-occurring conditions in autism and ADHD, and ADHD co-occurs in 50–70% of autistic people (Hours et al., 2022). These are further complexities to consider for the practitioner.

However, the enactive approach posits that cognition is not a solitary activity but one that emerges through dynamic interaction between autonomous systems – the therapist, the client, and their shared environment/the relationship (Lozada et al., 2024).

As emphasised in Chapter 12, it is crucial to understand how mental illness has historically been used as a tool for social control. We inherit a deep and damaging historical legacy, and greater awareness is required – especially where environmental and dominant societal values influence and condition what we define, describe and perceive as illness and wellness. This underlines the complexity of the presenting autistic client.

The traditional model of attunement may need to be rethought to bridge the relational gaps in order to foster a truly supportive relationship. Embracing and embodying one's own culture, in all its strengths, weaknesses and perpetual flux, requires a very high level of self-awareness.

Compounding the relationship is a fear among therapists and coaches of being seen by the patient/client as prejudiced or racist (Cowley, 2023), hindering transparency, thus blocking the authentic and empathic relationship needed for lasting healing and growth.

An enactivist philosophical perspective might help shift this relationship blockage. Ezequiel Di Paolo describes enaction as 'the ongoing process of being structurally and dynamically coupled to the environment through sensorimotor activity. Enaction brings forth an agent-dependent world of relevance rather than representing an agent-independent world' (Thompson, 2017).

This is explained more easily with the theory of Participatory Sense-Making (PSM) (De Jaegher & Di Paolo, 2007). PSM is situated within the enactive approach and is epistemologically very much aligned with Dialogue. It emphasises the co-creation of meaning through interaction by examined social interaction processes in subjectivity and intersubjectivity, examining the connections between how we interact and communicate together, and how we influence and understand each other and the world (together) and how all that makes us who we are.

In a therapeutic context, PSM is transformative as it shifts the focus from a hierarchical relationship – where the therapist is the expert and the client the passive recipient – to a more egalitarian model where both participants engage in mutual sense-making. This calls into question traditional power dynamics that often go unchallenged in therapy, particularly in settings where the therapist's expertise is prioritised over the client's lived experience.

Conventional therapies often operate from a normative framework that implicitly assumes a deficit within the neurodivergent individual. For example, cognitive-behavioural therapies (CBT) may unintentionally pathologise neurodivergent ways of thinking by labelling them as 'cognitive distortions'. The double empathy problem, as discussed by Milton (2012), highlights the disconnect where a 'neurotypical' therapist may struggle to fully understand the experiences of neurodivergent clients, leading to miscommunication and further marginalisation.

We can view the underlying principles of most therapy and coaching as dynamically 'agent-independent' – the cognition of both helper and helped are approached as independent of the system, as seen in the person-centred and relationship-centred approaches, and more obviously in a 'doctor–patient' style of helping, with its complex and far-reaching implications of power and dominance.

The relationship, however, is also a system, with its own autonomous life, and sensitive therapists will attest to the experience of witnessing the relationship 'being alive'. The enactive perspective views social interaction not as a secondary or auxiliary process but as central to how we experience and understand the world. In therapy, this implies that healing and change arise not solely from within the client or through the therapist's interventions but through the relational dynamics that both parties co-create.

A truly Dialogic approach would take this further by insisting on the recognition of the autonomous agency of all systems in the helping space. For the enaction principle to be active, and therefore generative change to take place, self-individuation of all systems must occur simultaneously, thus:

helped ↔ helping ↔ helper

Some therapeutic models lean more towards emphasis on helper–helped interaction processes. For example, Gestalt and Existential with their emphasis on 'here and now' and somatic observances. However, these do not consider the relevance of agency of all of the 'autonomous systems' in the room.

More work needs to be done towards building a comprehensive framework for engaging the enactive approach: 'This is the idea of dissolving barriers without erasing difference. In some cases, accepting boundaries but learning about the flows that cross them and how to see through them' (Di Paolo, 2022, para. 10).

Therapist and author Irvin Yalom expertly describes and embodies how being 'authentic and flawed for another flawed human requires bravery and a sense of safety' (Swanick, 2021). It is a deep level of vulnerability 'and reflexive awareness (or metacognition) which defines the helper as a person reflecting on her/his own role as he/she interacts' (Armstrong, 2012, p. 40), which allows deeper dialogue to occur and the desired outcomes achieved, whether they change or not.

A Dialogue approach to helping offers transformative potential, encouraging a shift from deficit-based perspectives to one of relational depth, authenticity, and equity.

AUTISTIC TRAUMA

In re-experiencing or reliving trauma during therapy, both the client and the therapist are engaged in a complex, co-created process. Vicarious trauma (Sultan, 2013) and client trauma transfer are commonly encountered in therapeutic work and are typically addressed in supervision. A Dialogic approach encourages a more nuanced understanding of trauma. Rather than focusing solely on the individual's trauma history, it emphasises the relational and systemic dynamics that contribute to the experience and perpetuation of trauma. An enactive approach would propose that this process involves more than just the reactivation of past trauma; it would also include the present relational dynamics, which, in the case of power imbalances from a dominant neurotype, may reinforce or exacerbate patterns of distress. If an autistic person has been told all their life that they don't communicate 'properly' and then a therapist highlights their 'faulty thinking' or suggests that difficulties with social interactions are 'irrational fears' about being judged, this could easily result in the recreation of past trauma or past deprivation in relationships. By focusing on the agency of all autonomous systems involved, a Dialogic approach would allow for a more holistic engagement with trauma – one that acknowledges its relational, embodied, and dynamic nature.

MASKING AND THE THERAPEUTIC PROCESS: THE ROLE OF INTERACTION

Non-autistic literature has presented masking as a social strategy – a way of getting by or fitting in in social situations (Cage & Troxell-Whitman, 2019; Tierney et al., 2016). More recently, autistic people describe how masking is not necessarily about appearing more normal or neurotypical, it is the trauma-fuelled projection of an acceptable and expected version of yourself to those around you that keeps you safe (Miller et al., 2021; Pearson & Rose, 2023). Masking could sometimes include the exaggeration of so-called 'autistic traits' depending on the context and expectations of those around the person. There are common misconceptions such as 'women mask better' or that 'men don't mask at all'. The celebration of 'behaving normally' by applauding autistics has been turned into social skills training and behavioural therapies with reward and punishment systems (Roberts, 2020). The amount of physical, emotional and mental energy that goes into masking is phenomenal and often leads to Autistic Burnout (Raymaker et al., 2020).

The concept of 'unmasking' refers to peeling away the layers of socially conditioned responses to reveal deeper, more authentic aspects of the self. Traditional therapeutic models often focus on symptom reduction, behaviour modification, or cognitive restructuring. A Dialogic approach shifts the focus to the interaction process itself. In Autism Dialogue, unmasking occurs not through the imposition of techniques but by facilitating an environment where the client's authentic experience can merge with it, and emerge organically, in relation to that conducive environment. This alludes to non-dual principles and because of the self-healing nature of the dialogic system, we can call it therapeutic.

As highlighted by Nic Higham (2023), a BACP Psychotherapist, Nondual Therapy emphasises direct engagement with the felt sense of experience, allowing clients to work with what is present, rather than resisting it. This approach, like Gestalt and others, aligns with the notion that therapy should not just aim to 'heal' or 'soothe' but to attend to the full spectrum of human experience, acknowledging both its challenges and its potential for growth.

DIALOGIC SUPERVISION

A Dialogue-informed approach to therapy would recognise the validity of neurodivergent perspectives and seek to deconstruct the normative assumptions embedded in traditional therapeutic models. It could be fruitfully used within group supervision contexts, where Dialogue is not merely a means of discussing cases but a method for exploring deeper questions around power, agency, and relational ethics. Questions such as 'Where am I, the facilitator, situated in this dialogue?' and 'How does societal power imbalance manifest in this space, right now?' would encourage therapists and supervisors to critically reflect on their positioning and the systemic forces at play.

Dialogue in groups extends beyond the mere exchange of ideas; it becomes a practice of collective sense-making. The goal is not to arrive at a consensus but to create a space where multiple perspectives, particularly those of marginalised or neurodivergent individuals, can be voiced and valued. This aligns with the broader enactive commitment to autonomy and relational depth, where the uniqueness of each participant is honoured without dissolving the differences that make each contribution valuable.

THE IMPORTANCE OF SAFE, NEURODIVERGENT-AFFIRMING THERAPEUTIC SPACES

Creating a safe and affirming environment is critical in an Autism Dialogue Approach (ADA)-informed practice. For neurodivergent clients, safety involves more than just physical or emotional security; it includes being free from the pressure to conform to neurotypical standards. Therapists must be aware of how therapeutic environments can either facilitate or inhibit the client's ability to engage authentically. Practical considerations, such as minimising sensory overload and respecting communication preferences, are essential for creating spaces where neurodivergent clients can feel truly understood and accepted.

ADA also emphasises the importance of the 'in-between' spaces in dialogue – the pauses, silences, and subtle shifts in energy that often carry as much meaning as the words themselves. Therapists are encouraged to focus on the quality of the interaction rather than simply on the content of what is being said. This requires a shift from a goal-oriented mindset to one that is process-oriented, allowing the therapeutic relationship to unfold naturally and in a way that honours the client's pace and needs.

The neurodiversity paradigm advocates viewing neurological differences as natural variations of human experience which challenges the dominant medical model that often pathologises neurodivergence (den Houting, 2019). Autism Dialogue goes further by integrating insights from intersectionality, recognising that neurodiversity does not exist in isolation but intersects with other axes of identity such as race, gender, and class. The therapeutic space often operates on normative assumptions rooted in white, Western cultural frameworks. Even well-meaning approaches that adopt a 'different, not deficient' stance may still perpetuate othering by positioning neurodivergence as a deviation from a presumed (fictional) norm. This issue becomes particularly evident in the treatment of autistic individuals, where therapies designed for neurotypical clients may inadvertently cause harm by reinforcing the very societal standards that marginalise them. Dialogue means a commitment to inclusivity, deconstructing assumptions and advocating for therapeutic practices that are not only neurodiversity-affirming, but also culturally responsive and intersectionality aware.

RELATIONAL HUMILITY AND THE PARADIGM SHIFT IN THERAPY

Relational humility is a key aspect of Dialogue, requiring helpers to acknowledge the limits of their knowledge and to approach their clients as people and with curiosity rather than certainty. This is particularly important when working with neurodivergent clients or those from marginalised communities. Traditional therapeutic models often prioritise the therapist's expertise, positioning them as the authority figure in the room. Dialogue, however, argues for a flattening of these hierarchies, recognising that the client's lived experience is an equally valid source of knowledge.

This shift requires a rethinking of what constitutes 'dysfunction'. In Autism Dialogue, dysfunction is reconceptualised as relational rather than individual. Rather than locating the problem within the client, ADA encourages therapists to consider how relational dynamics, societal structures, and systemic inequities contribute to the client's distress. This perspective aligns with critical disability theory and the social model that firstly views disability as a product of social constructs rather than a direct outcome of impairment. Second, it involves a complex interaction between an individual's impairment, their personal response to it, and the broader social context. Third, the disadvantages faced by disabled people stem from interactions between an individual's needs and societal barriers – whether physical, institutional, or attitudinal – that fail to accommodate them because they don't fit the traditional expectations of what is considered 'normal' (Hosking, 2008).

TRAINING AND IMPLEMENTATION: ADA AS A TRANSFORMATIVE PRACTICE

Given the rapidly diversifying social landscape, there is an urgent need for training programs that equip therapists with the skills to navigate complex cultural, neurodiverse and intersectional dynamics. ADA provides a comprehensive framework for such training, blending theory with practice in a way that is accessible and applicable to various therapeutic contexts.

Training in ADA involves not just intellectual understanding but experiential learning. Participants engage in reflective exercises, role-plays, and group dialogues that challenge them to confront their own biases, examine their positionality, and develop greater self-awareness. This process is designed to foster relational humility and to prepare therapists to engage more authentically and effectively with clients whose experiences differ from their own.

Moreover, ADA training emphasises the importance of ongoing learning and self-reflection. The goal is not to achieve a static state of competence but to cultivate a mindset of continuous growth and curiosity. By integrating ADA principles into their practice, therapists can create therapeutic relationships that are more equitable, responsive, and transformative.

CONCLUSION: TOWARDS A MORE INCLUSIVE AND RELATIONALLY ENGAGED THERAPEUTIC PRACTICE

The Autism Dialogue Approach represents a significant shift in how we think about therapy, moving from a focus on individual pathology and symptom reduction to a broader, more relational understanding of human experience. By integrating enactive theory, dialogic practice, and neurodiversity-affirming principles, ADA offers a pathway towards more inclusive, authentic, and effective therapeutic engagements.

In an era marked by increasing awareness of the importance of equity, diversity, and inclusion, ADA provides a timely and necessary framework for therapists, counsellors, and supervisors. It challenges us to rethink our assumptions, embrace relational humility, and commit to practices that honour the complexity and richness of human diversity. By doing so, we not only create more effective therapeutic spaces but also contribute to a broader societal shift towards greater understanding, acceptance, and compassion for all.

An upgrade in the underpinning philosophy, helping modalities and minds of professional helpers, towards a greater cultural self-awareness, is urgently required in order to effectively address the problems of our rapidly diversifying social landscape.

Professional helpers can be more dynamically aware, growing with clients towards better, more dynamic relationships of trust and responsibility, which is a paradigm shift away from a deficit approach, to one of deep embodiment, equity, social parity and abundance.

REFERENCES

Armstrong, H. (2012). Coaching as dialogue: creating spaces for (mis)understandings. *International Journal of Evidence Based Coaching and Mentoring*, 10(1), 33–47. Retrieved from https://radar.brookes.ac.uk/radar/items/6b2fdcb2-be2c-4f9c-8072-f48866aeb383/1/

Bader, M. (2009). The difference between coaching and therapy is greatly overstated. Retrieved from www.psychologytoday.com/gb/blog/what-is-he-thinking/200904/the-difference-between-coaching-and-therapy-is-greatly-overstated

Cage, E. & Troxell-Whitman, Z. (2019). Understanding the reasons, contexts and costs of camouflaging for autistic adults. *Journal of Autism and Developmental Disorders*, 49(5), 1899–1911. https://doi.org/10.1007/s10803-018-03878-x

Cowley, K. (2023). Own your identity. *Coaching at Work*, 18, 36–40.

De Jaegher, H. & Di Paolo, E. (2007). Participatory sense-making: an enactive approach to social cognition. *Phenomenology and the Cognitive Sciences* 6 (4):485–507. https://link.springer.com/article/10.1007/s11097-007-9076-9

den Houting, J. (2019). Neurodiversity: an insider's perspective. *Autism*, 23, 271–273.

Di Paolo, E. (2022). Enaction and dialectics – part 1. Retrieved from www.dialecticalsystems.eu/contributions/enaction-and-dialectics-part-i/#_ftn5

Ginapp, C. M., Greenberg, N. R., MacDonald-Gagnon, G., Angarita, G. A., Bold, K. W. & Potenza, M. N. (2023). 'Dysregulated not deficit': a qualitative study on symptomatology of ADHD in young adults. *PLoS One*, 18(10), e0292721.

Higham, N. (2023). What is non-dual therapy? Retrieved from https://nisargayoga.org/what-is-non-dual-therapy/

Hosking, D. L. (2008). Critical disability theory. Retrieved from www.lancaster.ac.uk/fass/events/disabilityconference_archive/2008/papers/hosking2008.pdf

Hours, C., Recasens, C. & Baleyte J. M. (2022). ASD and ADHD comorbidity: what are we talking about? *Front Psychiatry*, 13, 837424.

Kinnaird, E., Stewart, C. & Tchanturia, K. (2019). Investigating alexithymia in autism: a systematic review and meta-analysis. *Eur Psychiatry*, 55, 80–89.

Kiraz, S., Sertçelik, S. & Erdoğan Taycan, S. (2021). The relationship between alexithymia and impulsiveness in adult attention deficit and hyperactivity disorder. *Turk Psikiyatri Derg*, 32(2), 109–117.

Krishnamurti Foundation Trust. (n.d.). Regarding the quote 'It is no measure of health …' Retrieved from https://kfoundation.org/it-is-no-measure-of-health-to-be-well-adjusted-to-a-profoundly-sick-society/#:~:text=The%20nearest%20direct%20quote%20from,to%20make%20the%20individual%20unhealthy%3F

Lozada, M., Garcia, E., Chaoul, A. & D'Adamo, P. (2024). Towards an enactive approach to health: an integrative perspective which considers interdependence, agency, autonomy and participatory sensemaking in therapeutic phenomena. *Front. Psychol.*, 15, 1440751. https://doi.org/10.3389/fpsyg.2024.1440751

Miller, D., Rees, J. & Pearson, A. (2021). 'Masking is life': experiences of masking in autistic and nonautistic adults. *Autism in Adulthood: Challenges and Management*, 3(4), 330–338. https://doi.org/10.1089/aut.2020.0083

Milton, D. (2012). On the ontological status of autism: the 'double empathy problem. *Disability and Society*, 27(3): 883–887.

Paul, S. & Charura, D. (2015). *An Introduction to the Therapeutic Relationship in Counselling and Psychotherapy.* Sage. https://doi.org/10.4135/9781473909854

Pearson, A. & Rose, K. (2023). *Autistic Masking: Understanding Identity Management and the Role of Stigma.* Pavilion Publishing & Media Limited.

Raymaker, D. M., et al. (2020). 'Having all of your internal resources exhausted beyond measure and being left with no clean-up crew': defining autistic burnout. *Autism Adulthood*, 2(2), 132–143. https://doi.org/10.1089/aut.2019.0079

Roberts, J. (2020). Why perspective-taking and neurodiversity acceptance? Retrieved from https://therapistndc.org/why-teach-perspective-taking-neurodiversity-acceptance/

Siegal, D. J. (2011). *Mindsight: Transform Your Brain with the New Science of Kindness*. Oneworld Publications.

Siminovitch, D. E. & Van Eron, A. M. (n.d.). The pragmatics of magic – the work of gestalt coaching. Retrieved from https://potentials.com/2012/07/the-pragmatics-of-magic-the-work-of-gestalt-coaching

Sultan, N. (2013). Vicarious traumatization, burnout and self-care for mental health therapists: a literature review. *Academia*, 3, 26–35.

Swankick, R. (2021). The art of self disclosure: an ode to Dr. Yalom. Retrieved from www.musictherapyhere.com/post/the-art-of-self-disclosure-an-ode-to-dr-yalom

Thompson, E. (2017). The enactive approach. Retrieved from https://philosophyofbrains.com/2017/01/27/the-enactive-approach.aspx#:~:text=By%20%E2%80%9Cenaction%E2%80%9D%20we%20meant%20the,representing%20an%20agent%2Dindependent%20world.

Tierney, S., Burns, J. & Kilbey, E. (2016). Looking behind the mask: social coping strategies of girls on the autistic spectrum. *Research in Autism Spectrum Disorders*, 23, 73–83. https://doi.org/10.1016/j.rasd.2015.11.013

CHAPTER 15

Spirituality in Autism Dialogue

....

David Bohm's scientific exploration of interconnectedness points towards a profound, underlying oneness of the apparent multiplicity of the universe that transcends the apparent fragmentation of the world. For Bohm (1980), the universe is an undivided whole and separation is an illusion – the physical world (explicit) is a manifestation of a deeper, un-manifest (implicit) reality, always unfolding and enfolding in and out of each other. Bohm emphasised the transformative potential of recognising this unity, and that understanding the interconnectedness of all things could lead to a more harmonious and holistic approach to science, society and relationships.

The notion of the universe as self-organising suggests that the cosmos and all its components inherently move towards greater complexity and order without the need for external direction. In essence, this notion is reflected within the inner or esoteric dimension of most spiritual traditions and contrasts with traditional views of a mechanistic universe, where external forces like an external God drives change, which is another story for another day.

In nature and certain areas of organisational development, we know about regenerating/self-healing systems and group Dialogue is one such system, made up of individual human beings, who also in themselves contain mysterious qualities we conveniently describe as spiritual. Human Dialogue seeks to integrate social, scientific and spiritual worldviews, generating deeper insight and inviting a holistic understanding of reality (the context), to produce the right collective and individual actions.

In the 1980s Bohm turned to spiritual conversation with the Dalai Lama and J. Krishnamurti, and began conversations with public groups in England and the US. Notions of a new kind of dialogue began to emerge, and many deeply interesting video recordings of him from around this time are on the David Bohm Society YouTube channel. Evidently, Bohm was well under way to developing a dialogue practice influenced by much new spiritual understanding before he died.

NON-VIOLENT COMMUNICATION

As well as the many Dialogue approaches available to us, other approaches to communication particularly work for hyper-sensitive people as a personal framework for living, providing a more holistic way of life, which one might also consider as 'spiritual'.

One of these which very much aligns with Dialogue and a good example to briefly explore is Non-Violent Communication (NVC), developed by Marshall Rosenberg beginning in the 1960s (Rosenberg, 2003). NVC may resonate well with autistic people in terms of conflict who want clear and compassionate communication, or have a strong inclination towards introspection and inner peace. I recall one of my long-standing fears as a younger man was street violence and the ever-present possibility of being attacked by a group of men. Unfortunately, this seems more common in cities these days. NVC is a method of empathetic conversation that focuses on understanding and meeting the needs of both the speaker and the listener, expressed through four components – observations, feelings, needs, and requests. It states that although empathic connection fundamentally relies on connection at the level of feelings and needs, observations and requests may or may not be articulated. One can immediately see how this could be exacerbated by the 'double empathy problem'.

Autistic people struggle with identifying or expressing emotions in neuro-normative settings (Davis & Crompton, 2021). NVC provides a structured way to articulate feelings and needs, it can be empowering to help navigate social interactions more effectively. NVC emphasises clear, compassionate communication, which helps reduce ambiguity, making social exchanges more predictable and less stressful. It fosters an environment of mutual respect and understanding, which is crucial for the impact of feeling misunderstood or alienated in social situations. We can now develop this line of thought to include complementary spiritual practices and more intentionally peaceful ways of living life that are in line with dialogic perspectives.

SPIRITUAL COMMUNITY

Earlier in this book we explored how autistic communities need to be constructive and empowering rather than constraining and degrading (MacLeod, Lewis & Robertson, 2013). So-called spiritual communities also offer a sense of belonging and connection, crucial for reducing isolation and emphasising compassion, understanding, and acceptance. But we don't have to consider joining a monastic order or even a local meditation group. Teaching yourself, family members and caregivers peaceful communication techniques can improve the overall dynamics within the workplace and home, leading to a more supportive and nurturing environment. Schools and educators can benefit from incorporating these approaches to improve support for autistic students, creating a more inclusive and understanding atmosphere, where students are encouraged to express themselves and learn in ways that resonate with their uniqueness. In the workplace, promoting peaceful communication and understanding can help autistic staff thrive, thereby reducing misunderstandings and fostering a more inclusive and respectful work culture. What's a quiet room if it isn't for recovery and nourishment of the spirit? Autistic culture has evolved to use an energy currency called 'spoons', originally coined by Christine Miserandino (2003), which can be seen as a type of spiritual health measurement.

Mindfulness and meditation can help manage sensory overload, reduce anxiety and increase awareness of the present moment. Spiritual practices and a more peaceful lifestyle can support autistic people by providing a sense of grounding, inner peace, and connection to something larger than themselves. For example, many autistic people find solace in nature and with animals, where they can experience a sense of calm and connection. Engaging in activities like walking or playing in nature, gardening or simply spending time outdoors can provide a spiritual and peaceful retreat from the often overwhelming stimuli of daily life. Consider how our homes, once sacred bastions of peace, security and rest, are now too often dominated by various sizes of electronic windows out into the whole world.

SPIRITUAL PRACTICE AND THE INNER WORLD OF AUTISTIC PEOPLE

Rituals and routines can provide structure and predictability, which many autistic individuals find comforting to the spirit. Whether it's through daily meditation, prayer, or other spiritual practices, routines can help create a sense of stability and control in their lives. Rituals are less understood in autism, it's amusing when I see the word rituals used in the deficit frame, describing an autistic person's behaviour. I spent over 20 years practising rituals in a spiritual school, which gave me immense satisfaction and living inside a strict framework of life provided me with levels of freedom and insight that I've not experienced elsewhere. Perhaps on considering how people for thousands of years have lived ritualistically, we might consider leaning into that tendency for autistics instead of seeing it as a problem to be fixed or dissolved.

Olga Bogdashina is particularly known for her work on the sensory experiences and inner worlds of autistic people. She has also explored the connections between autism and spirituality, an area that has intrigued many but is less frequently discussed in mainstream discussions of autism. In her book *Autism and Spirituality: Psyche, Self and Spirit in People on the Autism Spectrum* (2013), Bogdashina argues that many autistic individuals have profound spiritual experiences or an innate spiritual awareness that is often overlooked or misunderstood. There are also a number of spiritual themes apparent in the writings of the authors mentioned below.

The heightened sensory experiences of autistic people can contribute to a deeper connection with the world around them; intense sensory experiences can be gateways to spiritual experiences and deep insight. This sensitivity can be intrinsically linked to an acute awareness of the interconnectedness of life, experienced as a spiritual or transcendent feeling and in the right environment, that sense of spiritual communion with others.

As autistic people perceive reality differently from most, altered perception can lend itself to spiritual or mystical experiences that challenge conventional understandings of spirituality and 'the world'. Autistic people often think in non-linear ways, which might allow them to access states of consciousness that are different from most other people; this could enable them to perceive reality in a way that aligns more closely with spiritual or mystical experiences.

William Stillman, an autistic author and speaker, has written extensively on the spiritual lives of autistic individuals. In his book *Autism and the God Connection* (2006), he argues that autistic people may have a unique spiritual connection that allows them to perceive and interact with the divine in ways that neurotypical people may not fully understand. Donna Williams, an autistic author and artist, has written about her spiritual experiences in her autobiographies, including *Nobody Nowhere* (1999a) and *Somebody Somewhere* (1999b). Williams describes her profound sense of connection to the world around her, often expressed through her art and music, and her feelings of existing in multiple realities or layers of consciousness. This relates to the concept of 'flow' and autistic monotropism. Temple Grandin, who is primarily known for her work in animal science, has also spoken about her experiences with spirituality on a podcast 'Inside the Mind of Temple Grandin' (Sounds True, 2016). Grandin, who identifies as an agnostic, has said that her sensory sensitivities and the way she processes information allow her to appreciate the mysteries of life and the universe in a way that feels spiritual, even if she does not subscribe to a specific religious belief.

The preference for solitude in many autistics is often seen as a fertile ground for spiritual growth and reflection. Many autistic people have rich inner lives and often engage in deep introspection, which, combined with solitude, can foster spiritual growth and a unique understanding of the self and the universe. Bogdashina (2013) notes that autistic people may have a different sense of self, one that is less bound by the ego and more connected to a universal consciousness. This perspective aligns with many spiritual traditions that emphasise the dissolution or 'taming' of the ego as enlightenment or awakening. It is generally accepted that autistic people are simply unable to conform to 'normal' standards of perception and therefore have to rely on intuition rather than information, making them more predisposed to monotropic depth and creativity. Twelfth-century Sufi Ibn Arabi said there is a distinction between formal knowledge of rational thought and the unveiling of insights into the nature of things (Stanford Encyclopedia of Philosophy, 2019), aligning with the autistic mind. Ibn Arabi contemplated the Logos, or 'Universal Man', as a mediation between the individual human and the divine essence. The notion of a universal prototype is interesting when we consider the philosophical conundrum of the mythical 'normal' standards of modern society. Modern thinking is largely focused on the level of material manifestation and cannot provide the deeper story required for human coherence. Michel Foucault described the inability of modernity to equip the individual with the necessary elements to be a whole, fulfilled human, saying that modernity lacked the 'technologies of the self' (Martin et al., 1988). To really complicate matters, Hallaq (2018) argues that using tools and concepts from within a paradigm to critique that paradigm is inherently limited. Aligning with Bohm's hypothesis of the restrictions of thought, Hallaq (2018) suggests that all modern knowledge systems are so deeply embedded in the structures of modernity that they cannot be useful in resolving modern problems.

Dialogue doesn't give in to normative logic and thought structures, and instead generates insight and intuitive knowledge, as a result of our sense-making – with love as the ground. As 'love is blind', Dialogue is a radical activity which aims to disturb and reorient. Group dialogue may thus cultivate a profound sense of unity and peace among participants. In my practice as a facilitator of group dialogue, I try to work at the very edges of meaning – as close to the edge as the group can safely get – constantly and gently enquiring. If there is to be a set agenda, it is of care and generosity and by clearing space for trust in what needs to emerge from the implicit, changes and shifts occur on the explicit.

So where does that leave us?

This broader perspective of dialogue underscores its significance in the implementation of a metaphysical and spiritual approach, which could be applied for enhancing spiritual, emotional, social and collective intelligence, and facilitating transformative change through regenerative processes, focussing on sustainability, resilience and fostering more flexible and adaptive organisational cultures.

I leave you with a verse from the Tao te Ching:

> Group process evolves naturally. It is self-regulating. Do not interfere. It will work itself out.
>
> Efforts to control process usually fail. Either they block process or make it chaotic.
>
> Learn to trust what is happening. If there is silence, let it grow; something will emerge. If there is a storm, let it rage; it will resolve into calm.
>
> Is the group discontented? You can't make it happy. Even if you could, your efforts might well deprive the group of a very creative struggle.
>
> The wise leader knows how to facilitate the unfolding group process, because the leader is also a process. The group's process and the leader's process unfold in the same way, according to the same principle.
>
> The leader knows how to have a profound influence without making things happen. For example, facilitating what is happening is more potent than pushing for what you wish were happening.
>
> Demonstrating or modelling behaviours is more potent than imposing morality.
>
> Unbiased positions are stronger than prejudice.
>
> Radiance encourages people, but outshining everyone else inhibits them.
>
> *(Tao te Ching, §58, 'Unfolding Process', trans. Heider, 2015)*

REFERENCES

Bogdashina, O. (2013). *Autism and Spirituality: Psyche, Self and Spirit in People on the Autism Spectrum.* Jessica Kingsley.

Bohm, D. (1980). *Wholeness and the Implicate Order.* Routledge & Kegan Paul.

Davis, R. & Crompton, C. J. (2021). What do new findings about social interaction in autistic adults mean for neurodevelopmental research? *Perspectives on Psychological Science*, 16(3), 649–653. https://doi.org/10.1177/1745691620958010

Hallaq, W. (2018). *Restating Orientalism: A Critique of Modern Knowledge*. Columbia University Press.

Heider, J. (2015). *The Tao of Leadership: Lao Tzu's Tao Te Ching Adapted for a New Age*. Green Dragon Books.

MacLeod, A., Lewis, A. & Robertson, C. (2013) 'Why should I be like bloody Rain Man?! Navigating the autistic identity. *British Journal of Special Education*, 40(1), 41–49.

Martin, L. H., Gutman, H., Hutton, P. H. & Foucault, M. (1988). *Technologies of the Self: A Seminar with Michel Foucault*. Tavistock.

Miserandino, C. (2003). The spoon theory. Retrieved from https://cdn.totalcomputersusa.com/butyoudontlooksick.com/uploads/2010/02/BYDLS-TheSpoonTheory.pdf

Rosenberg, M. (2003). *Nonviolent Communication: A Language of Life*. Puddledancer Press.

Sounds True. (2016). Inside the mind of Temple Grandin. Retrieved from https://resources.soundstrue.com/podcast/inside-the-mind-of-temple-grandin/

Stanford Encyclopedia of Philosophy. (2019). Ibn 'Arabî. Retrieved from https://plato.stanford.edu/entries/ibn-arabi/

Stillman, W. (2006). *Autism and the God Connection: Redefining the Autistic Experience through Extraordinary Accounts of Spiritual Giftedness*. Sourcebooks.

Williams, D. (1999a). *Nobody Nowhere: The Remarkable Autobiography of an Autistic Girl*. Jessica Kingsley.

Williams, D. (1999b). *Somebody Somewhere: Breaking Free from the World of Autism*. Jessica Kingsley.

CHAPTER 16

Resistance to change

....

Genuine dialogue means change is inevitable and requires individuals to confront differing viewpoints and engage in uncomfortable conversations. However, many people may shy away from such interactions due to a fear of conflict or a desire to avoid confrontation. In autism, there is the additional aspect of ongoing psychological and systemic oppression. I once heard an autistic person say, 'The last thing I need is dialogue.' Another said, 'The idea of sitting in a group scares me to death.' Fear can lead to a double empathy problem (Milton, 2012), surface-level conversations or a reluctance to engage in genuine dialogue about contentious issues.

Western societies have become increasingly polarised in recent years, with people identifying strongly with particular ideological, political, or cultural groups. This tribalism can create an 'us vs. them' mentality, making genuine dialogue difficult as people may be more focused on defending their group identity rather than engaging in open-minded conversation with those who hold different views. I think any movement can be self-alienating. I've met autistic people who puzzle me by wanting to enforce new social 'rules' about gender types and pronouns, and some who have scared me with a militant style of activism and sudden eruptions of suppressed rage.

With the rise of social media and personalised news algorithms, many people are exposed primarily to information that reinforces their existing beliefs and biases. This phenomenon creates echo chambers where individuals are insulated from diverse perspectives and may become resistant to engaging in dialogue with those who hold different opinions. While social media platforms offer opportunities for connectivity and communication, they also present challenges to genuine dialogue. Online interactions can be prone to misinterpretation, hostility, and polarisation, making it difficult to foster meaningful conversations that promote understanding and empathy.

In an era marked by scepticism and cynicism, there is often a lack of trust in institutions, media, and even fellow citizens, which can hinder genuine dialogue, as individuals may be reluctant to engage with others they perceive as adversaries or opponents. Additionally, a lack of empathy and understanding of each other's perspectives can further exacerbate social resistance to dialogue.

Western societies are grappling with deep-seated political and cultural divides, rooted in historical injustices, systemic inequalities or competing visions for the future. Overcoming such divides requires a willingness to listen, empathise, and engage in dialogue across ideological and cultural lines – a task that many find daunting or even impossible. Addressing social resistance to genuine dialogue in the West requires concerted efforts to bridge divides, foster empathy and create spaces for constructive engagement. Ultimately, building a culture of dialogue requires a collective commitment to listening, understanding, and engaging with one another in good faith.

AN AUTISTIC LEADERSHIP CULTURE

Generative Leadership means knowledge is created by those who are present in a *leaderful* environment (Raelin, 2011). By applying a set of easily learned skills, autistic participants make sense of a dynamic, microcosmic web of relationships, bringing self-empowerment, new social skills and less anxiety into their lives, families and the workplace. Non-autistic participants may identify as having privilege and make conscious changes in their lives and professions.

Right knowledge results in the right action and the dialogic process is iterative and practical. As knowledge emerges in situ, qualitative data gathering and reporting can become a streamlined process, co-designing and co-producing wherever possible. By providing opportunities and growing the cause, participants who build enough dialogue experience can emerge to become facilitators themselves.

'Valued leadership does not come from extraordinary people but from ordinary folk who remember what they know, recover their wits amidst the pressure of transitions and deal with what is immediate and present' (Williams et al., 2004, cited in Hawkins & Smith, 2013, p. 118). Consider a strengths-based authentic leadership approach for leadership development work and include *all* leadership (direct and indirect) to develop a leadership landscape that is inclusive and generative.

Changing a culture requires both the unlearning of old habits and the learning of new, and all members of an organisation look to the leadership team to see how it behaves (individually and collectively). It is therefore imperative that in an organisation, change starts with the top leaders setting direction, strategy and living the behaviours required to support and sustain the purpose and vision of the organisation.

Inclusion and belonging are essential elements to consider in any definition of culture and change. The change practices of Dialogue are rooted in powerful scientific theories, therefore extremely robust and unshakeable and continually shaped by those who engage. This is the implicit change principle in action and to demonstrate change occurs, you might work with what's known as warm data, a category of information specifically dedicated to 'transcontextual information about the interrelationships that integrate a complex system' (Bateson, 2017, para. 2).

The complexity of autism is evident across society, for example in the opposing views of the 'superpower' strengths-focussed, neurodiversity movement and the dominant paradigm of clinical and deficit models. As part of an inclusive organisational model, the best consulting process must be with those who are supported. 'Service-users' are seen as participatory stakeholders and should be fully included in processes. I would recommend a people's council, alongside the existing employees' group, which should be truly representative and integrated into strategy and operations.

Autistic people logically bring a broad range of direct experience including different language and communication styles, lived experience of countless nuanced traits and often unique and exceptional skill levels. As supporters, we have to learn from and assimilate these unique characteristics into our conscious lives and change our views of young people and those who do not speak and who have their lives ahead of them. Nurtured in an empowering dialogic environment a strong sense of self and social belonging will influence individuals, families and communities.

A leaderful autism environment creates a culture shift and deep social change that is urgently needed. Culture is the connecting pattern that pervades all elements of an organisation. A dialogic approach is uniquely placed to open our thinking around culture, to see the underlying beliefs and assumptions that influence 'how it is round here'.

Create a micro-community in your organisation, talking through sensitive and complex topics, whether they be personal, systemic or otherwise. Conversations should be facilitated by trained and experienced facilitators, who help break down barriers, increase cohesion and create a sort of fellowship that allows new insight and learning to emerge. The nature of dialogue is exploratory and part of an unfolding process; concepts such as diagnosis, intervention and other identifiers including autism itself, are deconstructed, which inevitably results in increased familiarity, enhanced social skills and reduction in psychological stress typically found in autistic people.

Different perspectives are held equally in Dialogue, and everyone aims to facilitate the best outcomes for themselves and the whole organisation. Participants learn and adhere to some simple practices, including slowing down normative modes of talking, for the group to build an atmosphere of trust and cohesion.

REFERENCES

Bateson, N. (2017). Warm data. Retrieved from https://norabateson.wordpress.com/2017/05/28/warm-data/

Hawkins, P. & Smith, N. (2013). *Coaching, Mentoring and Organizational Consultancy: Supervision, Skills and Development*. McGraw-Hill Education.

Milton, D. E. (2012). On the ontological status of autism: the 'double empathy problem'. *Disability and Society*, 27(6), 883–887.

Raelin, J. (2011). From leadership-as-practice to leaderful practice. *Leadership*, 7(2), 195–211. https://doi.org/10.1177/1742715010394808

APPENDIX 1

Case example: Autism Dialogue in Derby City and Derbyshire (England, UK)

....

In 2021 the Derby Clinical Commissioning Group (CCG) hired our firm, Dialogic Action CIC, to work with them to improve and develop their services for autism and neurodiverse communities. This case study describes and evaluates this piece of work; the study was co-produced by the stakeholders and participants in the project itself.

CCG faced several problems: specifically, they noted that their different services were fragmented, leading to a lack of coherence. Waiting lists were growing and people were 'falling through the net'. Parents, caregivers and children were suffering from a lack of support with knock-on effects to mental and physical illness, despondency and anger. The Clinical Group recognised that, over the long term, lack of appropriate provision was creating an unknown future, since today's neurodivergent young people are tomorrow's adults.

They also acknowledged that there are many existing (isolated) examples of good, enthusiastic initiatives but that staff, stakeholders and users who care were feeling disempowered and powerless because not all autism voices were being heard sufficiently. Derby CCG also appreciated that community is very important. The picture of service provision in January 2021 was a complex range of public-, private- and third-sector services that needed to demonstrate cost-effectiveness and success.

Dialogic Action CIC created the Autism Dialogue Approach with the aim of improving the lives of autistic people by tackling isolation, reducing social anxiety, raising acceptance, increasing community cohesion and addressing fragmentation in organisations. Our experience in this work has shown that including autistic people directly benefits them socio-therapeutically. Sharing stories, thoughts, and experiences of autism in a safe and confidential micro-community nurtures familiarity, reducing the negative effects of social anxiety that are increased by isolation. This approach raises morale, empowers people and leads to an improved sense of wellbeing and quality of life in a holistic, systemic fashion that benefits families and communities too.

To empower autism and neurodiverse communities and organisations, to facilitate and nurture a sense of belonging and empowerment. For example, help individuals and groups to become more reflective, offer peer group support and encourage self-help.

Their stated objectives made us a good fit to work together: to support communication universally, to renew empowerment of core staff and teams, to release systemic blocks and latent energy, to clarify common understanding and purpose, to revitalise both staff and clients, to improve health and wellbeing for staff and service users, to overhaul economics and save costs and, finally, to create a more dynamic, inclusive and accessible hub. We used dialogue to build towards these goals.

METHOD

Initial interviews

Before the dialogues we conducted nine individual interviews with the participants who were both stakeholders and leaders. We asked the following questions:

- If you look at the Derbyshire autism system today, what is your experience of it?
- If you could wave a magic wand, what would you change and how?

These interviews informed the two dialogue facilitators about how the prevailing system presented itself to the people using the services, and they provided improved understanding and relations with individuals in the cohort prior to the group work. Subtle characteristics of both individual and systemic influences were acknowledged by the interviewers, who were then better equipped as facilitators. The interviews were held in confidence; no feedback was provided to any other parties.

The Autism Dialogue format

A typical 'Autism Dialogue' on Zoom is usually up to 30 people and lasts from 90 minutes to three hours, including breaks. The number of sessions in a series varies from six to 10. Participants are consenting autistic adults (invited rather than referred), parents, workers and academics connected to autism. There should be a minimum of two experienced facilitators and one of them should identify as autistic (Asperger's included). Sessions open with a short, guided mindfulness session and, after a check-in, the group generates its own topics of enquiry and aims for slow-paced, free- flowing conversation using the four dialogic practices. It is a safe, confidential, and generative atmosphere, but not without discomfort. Silence is equally welcomed.

The sessions

We facilitated six two-hour generative 'Autism Dialogue' sessions (with up to 26 people) and a final thematic (non-Generative) session focusing on pulling together themes, which provided the opportunity for co-production of a report and recommendations, which was sent to the client.

OUTCOMES

This Dialogue series met the need for nurturing a sense of belonging and empowerment.

Participants reported that we need more conversations where we really listen: proper conversations. They also reported that Dialogue has heart, contrary to tokenistic meetings where decisions have already been made for autistic people. The group raised the importance of this kind of peer support and friendship, and how vital it is in the wake of diagnosis for autistic people to understand and accept themselves. Autistic people find solutions to problems through accessing the wisdom in the community rather than having to justify why something is a problem to begin with. There is an autistic need for freedom from the neurotypical (non-autistic) gaze, 'doing things our own way in our own time, without being excessively managed'.

LEARNINGS

Many people carry good intentions, but there is a lack of understanding, seen to be rooted in the pathological origins of autism. There is widespread confusion around terminology, with inappropriate and even harmful language and assumed power or expertise within the predominant neurotype. Services offer little or no support beyond diagnosis. Yet there is a desire for more autistic people to be meaningfully employed within the system, in such roles as mentors and counsellors, and a desire for specialist services.

Dialogue is seen as a supportive environment where neurodiversity can be celebrated and where people feel nourished. There is value of a dialogic approach in creating a sense of community between autistic and non-autistic people in Derbyshire, empowering seldom-heard voices to affect systemic change. There is positive impact on the wellbeing and personal growth of those attending the dialogues.

CONFERENCE SESSION EXTRACTS

Kate Salinsky: We were quickly asked to join in various meetings and to become part of the special educational needs strategy and discussion on what was needed for the system. We felt increasingly uncomfortable. Is this what we set out to do? One of our learnings was staying true to who we are and what we are doing and trusting the dialogue itself to do what dialogue does best. Bringing people together and allowing them to hear each other and to build together was the way that we were able to move forward. And it was very powerful for some of the commissioners of services to really hear what some of the autistic people were saying. This listening was made possible by the safe container we all created. It was extremely powerful, and also challenging at times. I think it left a big imprint in terms of the realization amongst those people about what they can do to make change.

Speaker: I do have a question. How did the participants partake? You had individuals that had autistic family members, and individuals that were actually autistic. So that's great but what's the dynamics of that?

Having a different scope of levels when it comes to the autistic individuals and not all individuals communicate effectively like we do. How was the scope? I'm trying to visualize it.

Jonathan Drury: There's an assumption that the less abled autistic people will not be in dialogue. We had dialogues where people have used AAC (augmentative and alternative communication machines) or had someone with them that can speak on their behalf – because they don't use the English language and use a different way of communication. But, generally, in the dialogues we run, people want to attend and use English as their spoken language. We make sure that we are clear with people that being part of the dialogue is simply being there, attending and listening with respect and suspension. If they are just listening, then that's fine. You are still as much of a part of the dialogue as when you are speaking. We ask people to have their video on as long as they're comfortable with it. If they're not, and quite often we see people turn their video on and off, it is generally because of sensory overload and they need to quiet down. The breadth of what's acceptable is much wider and because of that people are comfortable to express themselves.

Speaker: The comfort of being yourself. I love that. I have worked with autistic students for years and have been trying to find a way to let them know that it's okay to be yourself – especially when you have sensory sensitivities. So I just want to say thank you for that. I've never put it that way even though I have years of working with different individuals.

The comfort of being yourself – that's what it's all about. Bringing in dialogue just to make them comfortable in groups and able to talk and communicate. I loved reading the paper as it helped me find really useful ways to change the dynamic of a situation.

Speaker: I have a lot of neurodiverse people in my life for various reasons. Yesterday I was giving a Covid vaccine, and I realized pretty quickly that the person I was administering the vaccine to was not neurotypical. I don't know her diagnosis, we didn't talk about it, but she was really very nervous about needles, which is a separate issue from her being neurodiverse. But her expression of not wanting to have a shot was different than what my expression might have been. I found myself wondering what to do in this situation. I was doing my best to keep her calm and say, 'You don't have to do this'. I was trying to do grounding things with her to see if that helped and asking her what she needed, but she was in a place where she couldn't even respond to me. We ended up getting through it by her putting on headphones and listening to music. It would've been pretty interesting if we had a framework of dialogue that helped us to talk to one another. We didn't, and there's no societal structure set-up where she and I can move into a mode of dialogue allowing us to talk to one another. So we did the best we could. We got through it, and she was okay and I was okay, and everything was fine. But in that meeting with the commissioner, it would be really interesting for them to hear about a shared framework of dialogue. I just applaud you all for using dialogue in such a useful way. Altering life for people, which this should be about, rather than checking a box.

Speaker 2: That's a brilliant way to finish the session.

POSTSCRIPT

These are the author's reflections, written some months after the conference.

One participant from Derby attended Autism Dialogues in Sheffield for two years, which then resulted in an introduction being made to the right person within their local authority, who had the open-mindedness to listen and understand, and the power to make something happen. This organic human process is as much a part of dialogue and its proliferation as the initial felt-sense, years previously, that there are people out there who desperately need dialogue. Personal contacts and professionalism are required to create the trust that's needed in this field at a systemic level, in order to give way to the impersonal and generative. A good chemistry between both leadership teams carried through and the required final report was edited for this paper, as a matter of course.

One thing our small team didn't anticipate was the confusion that came at us from several elements of the system – including parents who seemed angry and almost hostile and consultants with complex agendas – and each took equal amounts of effort to unravel ourselves from. As the extract shows, we the facilitators quickly grew a heightened awareness, and once attuned to these fault lines it's almost like a managed trauma. When similar language was used in the conference presentation, such as one person saying, 'not all individuals communicate effectively like we do', our language-awareness spotlights the privilege of the predominant neurotype. Facilitators are like the canaries in the coal mine – a phrase also commonly used in relation to the very high sensitivity of autistic people.

It was a powerful learning experience for me, the team and reportedly most of the participants. It has made my vision sharper and, without lasting damage, increased my resilience and professionalism. As I write this, I have the image of walking into the middle of a raging battlefield and laying down a red rose, which I hope has taken root, and whose scent is picked up by the right people.

ACKNOWLEDGEMENT

This appendix is reprinted from J. Drury, K. Salinsky & J. Elliott (2022) Autism Dialogue in Derby City and Derbyshire. In H. Wagener & C. Penwell (eds), *The World Needs Dialogue! Four: Putting Dialogue to Work* (pp. 83–88). Dialogue Publications. Reproduced with permission.

APPENDIX 2

Case example: community online series 2022

....

This project (carried out in 2022 during a COVID-19 lockdown in the UK) aimed to foster connection, inclusion and understanding among autistic people, their families and professionals through a national series of six Autism Dialogue sessions on Zoom. During lockdown, where the situation for autism community was on the whole getting worse, it was important for Dialogica to offer a unique, socio-therapeutic space designed to reduce isolation and anxiety. We aimed to enable safe, authentic, and equitable conversations between autistic and non-autistic participants using the approach. Delivered over six months, the programme included taster sessions, two dialogue series guided by experienced facilitators, and follow-up events, attracting a diverse mix of attendees. Feedback revealed significant benefits, including a strong sense of belonging, reduced masking, and improved wellbeing. Participants emphasised the value of shared understanding, safe participation, and the unique opportunity for growth the dialogues provided. The sessions also inspired ongoing peer-led support groups, highlighting a powerful and unexpected ripple effect. Key lessons include optimising group size, enhancing evaluation methods, and improving administrative systems to support future expansion.

1. BACKGROUND

1.1 What we set out to do

A grant of £9850 was given by The National Lottery Community Fund – Awards for All to host a national monthly series of six 'Autism Dialogues' on Zoom to help up to 50 autistic people, parents, carers, teachers, and healthcare professionals.

1.2 What is the Autism Dialogue Approach?

Autism Dialogue is socio-therapeutic participatory action research that benefits individuals and their communities. The approach is particularly suited to autistic people because of the attention to processing time and the space given between speaking, and because it is a safe, confidential system that relies on everyone's generosity and care. Sharing stories, thoughts and experiences in a safe, confidential setting nurtures familiarity and reduces the negative effects of social anxiety that are increased by isolation.

1.3 What was delivered and how

We held an initial online seminar and 'taster session' in March which 25 people attended. Then, between April and October 2022 Dialogica hosted two dialogue series (Group A and Group B) which were four sessions of 2.5 hours each. The conversations were guided by two experienced facilitators. Attendees were a mixture of autistic and non-autistic people, parents, carers, and professionals. For group A attendance varied across the four sessions from between 12 to 20 people. Similarly in Group B the attendance varied between 7 and 15 people.

2. WHAT DIFFERENCE DID AUTISM DIALOGUE MAKE TO THE COMMUNITY?

2.1 Feedback

We sent out a Google forms evaluation after each series with some questions. Additionally, after the Dialogues concluded we held two follow-up events at which we gathered feedback. One was an online event, followed the next day by a smaller in-person local dialogue event in Sheffield with an optional social element. This allowed people to choose the event which best met their preferences. Below is a summary of the feedback grouped by theme.

Theme 1: Safe, supported, included

It was felt by many that the facilitators created a safe container which enabled participation through gently holding the space and sharing power with attendees.

> *'I liked that all were involved and the facilitator would get others involved so not only the few would be heard. I was very happy that there was so many opinions so I could go away and think over what was discussed then I was able to figure out what was best for me.'*

> *'The facilitators helped to create a calming, welcoming space. I appreciated that there was no sense of "them and us".'*

Theme 2: 'Challenging but good'

The sessions were not without challenge for many participants however this was perceived as valuable and an opportunity for growth, rather than being overwhelming.

> 'At times I felt "out of it" as someone who is not autistic, but that in itself was good to experience!'

> 'Challenging, insightful, provocative (in a good way), mind expanding, tiring, clarifying, safe enough to "try to" take risks.'

Theme 3: Belonging and connection

A number of participants expressed how they quickly felt accepted and a sense of belonging within the group. This was important to people as they rarely experienced this in other settings.

> 'Thank you everyone. Joining a collective space is so meaningful for me. I appreciate all of you.'

> 'These sessions have reminded me that I'm not alone in my experience and struggle.'

> 'The thing that surprised me the most, in a really good way, was how rapidly a sense of community developed within the group. The shared experience of autism/neurodiversity created such a rapid sense of belonging and also an urgency to share experience finding yourself in a space where you were understood.'

Theme 4: Authenticity

Participants strongly appreciated the autism dialogues as a safe space where they felt they could be more their authentic selves.

> 'The only place where I cannot mask – a place where I am "me".'

> 'A place where I can practise trying not to mask – a safe, non-judgemental space. Testing out talking without the mask – but it's still challenging. Have masked for nearly 60 years so it is still very anxiety provoking coming out from behind the mask.'

> 'I feel accepted – autistic or not – without having a definite label for myself.'

Theme 5: Equity across neurotypes

Overall participants valued the unique bringing together of NT and Autistic people in one supportive space.

> 'There is space for both autistic and non-autistic people and the dialogue addresses concerns that are universally shared.'

'Different neurotypes can learn from each other I came to learn more about my son. I've learned so much through people sharing.'

'I don't know what the social rules are – I like it when NTs can explain it to me in the group.'

Theme 6: We want more!

There was a strong, consistent message from all the feedback gathered that people wanted opportunities to participate in further dialogues.

'There isn't anything like this anywhere else. So more sessions would be valued.'

'We feel like friends – I feel like I belong and this is why I enjoy it – it's meeting up with friends in a comfortable space. When it stops it feels like losing friends.'

2.2 Impact

We asked participants to complete 'before and after' zoom polls. Responses showed:

- Improvements in areas of belonging, acceptance of self, feeling accepted by others, feeling connected and happy.
- Reductions in feeling distressed, anxious, guilty or ashamed.
- 86% said they would strongly recommend Autism Dialogue to others and 14% said they would recommend it (so 100% would recommend).

2.3 Added Value: Autism Dialogue Friends Group

Some of the participants found they had enough in common to continue an informal group of their own via Zoom and a WhatsApp group which is called Autism Dialogue Friends. The group has met nine times so far and generated approximately 102.5 hours of support to date (20.5 hours of meetings with an average of five attendees per meeting). This is a very satisfying outcome, which we didn't expect. More information on these groups can be found in a separate summary report.

3. LESSONS LEARNED

- Group size of 12 to 15 is optimum.
- We can expect some dropout as people will try it but some will decide its not for them.
- More systematic evaluation is required – such as using validated scales before and after the dialogues.
- Improved admin and record keeping systems will be important to support our expansion.

4. WHAT'S NEXT?

- We want to offer regular autism dialogues and are exploring funding possibilities to support this.
- We are developing facilitator training to increase the capacity of Dialogica to deliver more autism dialogues and enable practitioners to use the approach in their own work.
- We are exploring partnerships and funding to support more robust evaluation and to understand more about the processes within autism dialogue that benefit our participants.
- In August 2023 we signed a contract with a major publisher for *The Autism Dialogue Approach Handbook* [i.e. the present volume] to be released in 2024.

APPENDIX 3

Case example: post-dialogue group community – 'Autism Dialogue friends'

BACKGROUND

After taking part in Dialogue Group B (four two-and-a-half-hour sessions), several group members were keen to continue meeting to maintain the sense of belonging and shared experience they gained from the dialogue group. This was headed by one particular individual who had found the sessions incredibly beneficial and did not want the connection to end abruptly. This led to interested individuals agreeing to share their email addresses and subsequently their mobile numbers to allow a WhatsApp group to be set up.

WHATSAPP GROUP – 'AUTISM DIALOGUE FRIENDS'

The WhatsApp group was initially set up to arrange meetings but has become a safe space for the group to share and have asynchronous discussions between meetings. It has now (as of July 2023) been running for eleven months with no sign of it ending anytime soon. One member of the group does not have WhatsApp, so information about meetings is shared with them via email.

MEETINGS

Meetings are online and follow the same principles as dialogue sessions but are self-moderated. One group member provided 'gentle facilitation' for the first two meetings, but after this the group decided it was not necessary. There is still a guided mindfulness at the start of the session led by willing group members and a ten-minute break half-way through. It was also decided early on that formal check-ins and check-outs weren't needed due to the size and informality of the group. Meetings were initially arranged by voting in an online poll, but more recently the group has agreed to meet every four weeks, 5.30 to 7.30 p.m., on a Saturday, to make things simpler.

FACTS AND FIGURES

- There are eight members of the group, seven of whom are part of the WhatsApp group.
- Over four hundred messages have been shared on the WhatsApp group.
- The group has met nine times to date (July 2023) with the intention to continue meeting monthly for the foreseeable future.
- Four meetings have lasted two hours, and five meetings have lasted two and-a-half hours.
- On average five group members have attended each meeting.
- The meetings have therefore generated approximately 102.5 hours of support to date (20.5 hours of meetings with an average of five attendees per meeting).

QUOTES FROM GROUP MEMBERS

- 'I felt a deep connection to the people in my dialogue group and was keen to keep this going. The informal meetings we have arranged have kept those connections going and provided support at difficult times, especially the demands and expectations of Christmas.'
- 'For me it is a safe space where I'm able to share my feelings and discuss the issues that are getting me down. A group of friends who listen and support each other, who are there with advice and are non-judgemental about the issues you are experiencing.'
- 'I feel more at ease in the group than I feel in most other social situations.'
- 'It feels like everyone in the group understands fully the fundamentals of the dialogue method. That I think is important for the talks to function so well.'
- 'I'm thankful to have an ongoing developing group stemming from the dialogues which provides a rare sense of belonging and shared understanding where we can gently develop within it as our authentic selves and discuss shared issues in a safe space.'

Thanks to Nick Russell for writing this report.

APPENDIX 4

Case example: Autism Dialogue coaching

....

I am fortunate to have a level of hyper-empathy, which I've learned to channel into dialogic coaching and group dialogue facilitation. My one-to-one coaching of non-autistic executives (working in the autism field) has been successful as well as with autistic people. Overall, whether autistic or not, I am aiming to cultivate an environment with an improved sense of presence, which is safe and comfortable for the client who can slowly introduce their version of reality and with whom I can engage in; 'co-creation is this beautiful experience where two worlds meet. Where the therapist gets to experience a part of the client's reality and consequently the client can experience the presence of another in this co-creation.' (Bonnici, 2020, pp. 6–7). I'm not a therapist but the word coach can replace the word therapist here, so it has the intended meaning, whilst I ask you to recall the initial recovery elements of dialogic coaching for autistic people in seeking to move forward in their lives. Again, we return to the power of the Dialogic environment for transformation and healing, which regeneration and leadership consultant Katherine Long described to me thus:

> Presence-based dialogue is an alchemical process, turning ordinary listening skills into a channel for deep, felt sense connection to the shared ground of being, supporting the unfolding of new meanings and ideas. Knowing how to cultivate the conditions for this kind of dialogue is the defining hallmark of a truly transformational coach.
>
> *(Katherine Long. personal communication,*
> *30 September 2024)*

Below is a brief outline of what I can call Autism Dialogue Coaching, with a vignette of a case with an autistic person, followed by a few pointers I hope you find useful. There is another short case study below that.

Dialogic coaching isn't yet fully defined (although this book is about the Autism Dialogue Approach and in the group sense has some alignments with what's called group coaching). For the purposes of framing and having a better understanding of something called Autism Dialogue Coaching, we can situate it within Gestalt, which has inherent aspects of existentialism, relational theory, engagement theory and love, much of which I have already covered within Dialogue.

> Dialogue is the basis of the gestalt therapy relationship. In dialogue, the therapist practices inclusion, empathic engagement, and personal presence, e.g. self-disclosure. In the process of doing this, the therapist confirms the existence and potential of the patient, the therapist imagines the reality of the patient's experience and in doing so confirms existence of the patient.
> *(Yontef & Jacobs, 2005, p. 320)*

Gestalt/Dialogic coaching is coaching in the here and now. It involves deep, authentic self-enquiry, asking yourself 'Can I trust this, right now, in its entirety?' Below I describe an experience using a specific Gestalt method known as 'use of self':

I pointed out the client's fingers drumming on the chair, which resulted in a burst of surprised laughter, opening a door of trust between us. This was an interesting reaction, from my spontaneous but conscious intervention, that could've been taken the wrong way and showed me the trust was building. The client followed with a flow of mining their own inner landscape, while asserting their values and care for others but also, in their work as a skilled craftsperson, around using natural materials and sustainable methods. This was a powerful association and included their use of a strong house as a metaphor.

At one point they said, 'I've been busy forever', which made me feel quite sad and tired myself and I even felt heaviness in my chest and tears come to my eyes. I told the client this and that I was also surprised at the reaction their remark caused in me.

I like to think of Dialogue as the vehicle in which a coach and client travel, so that they unfold their own story together as well, driving along, whilst the client is supported to explore their narrative. Each takes turns with the wheel. The coach's work is to enhance perception of the micro-elements of the driver, the passenger and the journey, moment by moment.

Engaging with others' stories offers us an aesthetic and relational lens rather than a 'scientific' or rational lens through which we can understand people's behaviours, values, beliefs and attitudes.

Clients are encouraged to unfold and build on their past, present and future by telling authentic stories and we both slowly move towards understanding these profoundly through dialogue. Over time, their reflection deepens by exploring the narratives and are supported to develop critical insight and appreciate their stories through analysis of them.

In the 'vehicle' of Dialogue, as we travel along together, growing in trust, clients gradually learn that all of our pasts are 'in' our present and they were previously unaware of this. We all learn to get on with our lives, but without enough awareness, the past will confront our present in unhelpful ways. Coaching sessions can become occasions where the past is brought usefully into the present and interwoven into their future hopes, dreams, visions and goals. This process is underneath what is meant by discovery in coaching; the client discovers a more helpful and satisfying way of telling their stories and discovers new perspectives that frame the desired future in better ways.

EMPATHY AND USE OF SELF

Perhaps an extreme example of hyper-empathy is once when I had an acute stabbing discomfort in my chest immediately before a client said they had some bad news about their own breathing difficulties. The use of self is when the coach uses their own experience of being with the person as data and communicates this to the client to deepen their awareness. This experience may be bodily experiences, feelings and images that come to mind. When considering the use of self the coach has to weigh up whether an intervention is likely to facilitate the client, and how to say it in a way that is likely to be received usefully to them. Empathy relates to mutual understanding and high levels of awareness, but is it more than that? Self-reflection is key to a good level of empathy, yet, like trust, it cannot be artificially created.

LISTENING

Some of the basics of good listening include paraphrasing, which is listening to the client and then putting back to them the meaning of what was said, in your own words. Summarising is an extended form of paraphrasing, playing back to the client the information, themes and issues that have been spoken about over a longer period. Noticing their body language and themes emerging in stories and language. All of this is part of the Dialogue process – listening is one of the four dialogue practices and is covered more fully in Chapter 5.

DISCONNECTION

Moments of disconnection might occur when a sense of direction is lost, when you lose rapport or when the conversation loses energy. At these times you can accept that some problems are insoluble, so trust your intuition, hold the silence (one of my favourites) or discuss the disconnect openly. Remember, autistic people usually appreciate frank authenticity, and why not? So you're feeling awkward or uncomfortable – tell them. You don't know what's happening – tell them. This way you're instantly empowering your client and building an authentic relationship, which is why they're there.

Think about how you develop and embed empathy, gestalt and dialogic presence in your coaching practice.

SOME QUESTIONS

- What issues do you face?
- Are you aware of context switching and additional pressures on autistic people in the workplace?

A question for your new autistic coachee in a leadership role might be:

- How does your unique way of thinking and processing information shape the way you approach challenges at work, and how might you leverage this strength to lead more effectively?

AUTISM DIALOGIC COACHING – SHORT CASE STUDY (IDENTIFYING FEATURES CHANGED)

Rachael, a 35-year-old autistic woman, approached me seeking support for her struggles with social isolation and communication challenges. Over five one-hour sessions, we applied the Autism Dialogue Approach, focusing on creating a safe, supportive space for her to explore her experiences without pressure.

At the outset, I introduced the four core dialogue practices – voicing, respect, suspension, and deep listening – and explained how they could help shape our conversations. Rachael was receptive, expressing an interest in applying these practices as she saw fit. Each session began with either a short guided mindfulness exercise or a period of shared silence. Rachael usually chose the guided version, though once she opted for two minutes of quiet, sitting together with our eyes closed.

In the first session, Rachael opened up about her lifelong struggle with social anxiety and the fear of being misunderstood. She often felt pressured to conform to conventional communication norms, which left her feeling disconnected from her true self. The dialogue space, grounded in deep listening, allowed her to voice these concerns without judgement.

By the second session, Rachael became more comfortable with the natural pauses and moments of 'suspension' in our conversations, where we held our assumptions lightly. This created a slower, more intentional pace that gave her the time to reflect on her emotions and bodily sensations. In these moments, there was a sense of 'gestalt presence' – a kind of holistic awareness that emerged as we focused on the 'here and now.' This presence allowed Rachael to become more fully attuned to herself, heightening the depth of the dialogue and creating a powerful atmosphere and connection as everything seemed to bond.

In sessions three and four, Rachael's confidence grew. Through the practice of authentic voicing, she began to reframe her experiences, recognising that her discomfort in social situations was often a response to societal expectations, rather than a personal flaw. The magic of gestalt presence continued to play a role in deepening her awareness, helping her understand her preferences and communication needs in a more integrated way.

By the final session, Rachael reported a newfound sense of agency in her interactions. The Dialogue process, supported by mindfulness and the felt sense of presence, had helped her embrace her unique ways of being, allowing her to connect more authentically with herself and others.

REFERENCES

Bonnici, J. (2020). Gestalt therapy and autism: a possible symbiotic relationship. Retrieved from www.academia.edu/43325739/Gestalt_Therapy_and_Autism_A_Possible_Symbiotic_Relationship

Yontef, G. & Jacobs, L. (2005). Gestalt therapy. In R. J. Corsini & D. Wedding (eds), *Current Psychotherapies* (7th ed., pp. 299–336). Thomson Brooks/Cole Publishing.

APPENDIX 5

Case example: an encounter

....

By way of story, I provide an account of an informal and, for me, very powerful and positive dialogic encounter with an autistic man who I was supporting. I include it here to illustrate how dialogue takes place all around us all the time, in the same way I've included the description of my brother's demise and consequent passing as a result of lack of dialogue. I hope you appreciate these examples and their very different natures within the pervasive and elemental nature of dialogue.

>Life by its very nature is dialogic.
>
>*(Bakhtin, 1984, p. 293)*

On the first day of a new job, I stood waiting nervously in the carpeted lounge, trying to act casual. I was to be supporting a young autistic man in his family home, with no training or experience, and on this preliminary visit, his parents briefed me before disappearing. A long minute later James suddenly appeared, closed the door behind him, holding his left hand out, in a loose fist, looking me directly in the eyes, with a kind and warm expression from under a hoodie.

'Hello, Jonny.'
'Hello, James.' I softly held his fist.
The atmosphere became empathically alive, and I felt cared for. The front of his hoodie was pulled up, revealing his portly stomach, which he kept looking down at and patting. I wondered, was he doing this to divert my attention away from his face, or nothing so conscious? We stood facing each other, like new friends, with what we had in common as yet unknown. His dad's head appeared round the door. 'Excuse me, Jonny, would you like a tea, we've got mint?'
'Oh mint, yes please.'

'Mint tea, yes, mint tea,' James echoed in a high and wistful voice, turning to look through the large window onto the snow-covered street. Now cupping my tea, I sat down on the sofa, highly curious in anticipation.

Without turning round, James asked, 'What were you like as a child, Jonny?' His parents had said he would ask questions about me for about ten minutes and then tell me to go, so I remained vigilant.

I explained to him how I was mostly happy as a child, but didn't have many friends.

'Why do you think you didn't have many friends?' I noted his theme continuing.

'Because I wasn't really interested in most people.'

I continued talking about my youthful troubles then suddenly sensed it was too much.

'Oh, I don't do any of that,' James said.

I asked what he was like when he was younger.

'I don't know … I don't know.'

I thought I heard an ounce of a crying tone in his voice, a sort of deep cry of aloneness and detachment from this world …

'I don't know …' I quickly discovered, would be his immediate answer to most questions, followed sometimes by an answer, but still, it seemed like an effort for him to put words together, and taught me not to ask too many questions. James continued to stare out of the large window, forehead occasionally touching the glass, belly on display to the neighbours to whom I imagined it providing something of a diversion in this quiet and reserved neighbourhood.

As I watched him, I realised James was fully aware of the moment, and I was with him, we were connecting. I had an acute sense of it, which gave me a spacious sensation, but the price for him of this hyper-awareness was deep, existential struggling. Unprepared for this world, heavy with its concepts, restrictions, expectations and old stories, a child or adult living fully, unwittingly in the moment is poor in survival skills. Something in me wanted to know him personally by talking, but why, when I knew it would cause him stress? When I continued with his own topic, he would say, 'Yeah that as well … that as well' as if he was vocalising immediacy, in the workings of his mind; Like 'Yes, Jonny, so you are now adding more words to my experience …' Keeping more and more quiet for us, I felt a sudden flash of awareness of the unique man in front of me, contrasting sharply with years of accumulated information in the formal studying of autism.

'Do you know any celebrities?' He came and sat on a chair near me, squeezing his naked belly. We now talked about music. I learned he has singing lessons and to my surprise, he sang for me a few heartfelt words from 'Another Brick in the Wall'. I almost sang along.

Our mostly comfortable silences were getting longer between the chatter.

Silence and space were of equal importance to the verbal and physical aspects of our connection.

I felt a certain reverence, for here was someone who was not of this world, which made this both personal and impersonal. There was the sensation I was in the presence of a cosmic phenomenon, an ethereal mystery, which moved me.

At the same time, in the context of becoming his potential carer, here was a struggling person.

Nonetheless, James was a human who had already, perhaps long ago, by omission of norms, had an elevation of being, that state of pure release that perhaps is driving everyone and everything about being human. There wasn't an idolising on my part, but rather a unification with a common soul.

James had something incredibly important to impart to me and the world, something so raw and so honest about this being human.

'I think I'll go when I've drunk this,' I offered.

'Go. Yes. OK, that's fine.' And he was gone first, out of the door.

Sitting now by myself for a minute, cup still in hand, I felt the room quiver around me in response to our meeting.

On the way home as I reflected, feeling quite emotional, and resting later, behind my closed eyes I had the sensation of floating in space, and there with me was James.

REFERENCE

Bakhtin, M. M. (1984). *Rabelais and his World*. Indiana University Press.

APPENDIX 6

A note on research and evaluation

Key to understanding how we approach generative dialogue are the concepts of evaluation and research and participation.

Evaluation is derived from the Greek meaning of value or strength. A certain value or strength is set, to which further iterations of a model are measured against, therefore seeking to maintain that original standard or value; strength, power and the status quo of existing structures is maintained by measuring further examples against that value proposition.

Dialogue is a dynamic human process, whose tools of thought and language, our fundamental means of communicating anything, don't have an implicit value standard, therefore aren't measurable by typical means.

Sociological theories have yet to significantly influence values-led activities, but by applying phenomenological concepts, for example, we can reveal the limitless potential for creativity – challenging and transcending our assumed social structures and constraints. Phenomenology posits that individuals possess a shared knowledge base that forms their reality, a reality taken for granted and learned through social interaction. Shared knowledge creates the assumption that everyone experiences the same world, but what we perceive as real is not inherently so.

Understandably, dialogue hasn't yet been formulated as a research model in and of itself.

PARTICIPATORY RESEARCH

In 2018 a group of ten individual autism researchers reflected on their own series of seminars, stating:

> Specific manifestations of participatory research might include leadership by autistic researchers, partnership with autistic people or allies as co-creators of

knowledge, engagement with the community in general (e.g. via social media) and consultation with relevant individuals or community organisations.

(Fletcher-Watson et al., 2018)

There needs to be a clear understanding of what 'specific manifestations' means, how these come about and into what atmosphere. While seemingly based on equity design and cohesive, participatory research, a problem with the approach suggested is that it is very much led from the top, where the final outcome is that self-appointed experts (certain academics and invited individuals) tell others how they should and shouldn't do research. For example, who decides who is appropriate as 'leadership' or 'allies' and who decides what are 'relevant individuals or community organisations'? Autistic researcher Michell Dawson elaborated on the implications in a tweet:

> Promoters of 'participatory' research erase the diverse interests & contributions of most autistic researchers (past & present) … There are many autistic researchers with diverse interests & work. Most are excluded from the 'participatory' research literature, where only on-message autistics are allowed.
>
> *(Dawson, 2018)*

Fletcher-Watson et al. (2018) continue: 'materials to enable this burgeoning community of practice to extend and improve their work, and specifically to include a wider diversity of autistic perspectives, remain lacking'.

Research methods such as Interpretative Phenomenological Analysis (IPA), which work more directly with experience, need to be aligned with Dialogic modalities. To conduct an IPA study, researchers must engage in a double hermeneutic, a process whereby the researcher tries to make sense of the participant trying to make sense of what is happening to them, so IPA could be an appropriate implementation for exploring more accurate representations of participation. IPA is underpinned by theory which looks at both phenomenology, where a person's subjective experience of a particular phenomenon is examined, and heuristics which looks at how people understand and make sense of their experiences. IPA is potentially useful for gaining an insight into the lived experience of autistic individuals and aligns well with participatory approaches. From enactivist and dialogic perspectives, however, the 'researcher' isn't apart from the participant – they are inextricably bound. Grounded theory, action research, authoethnography and other research methods will all require a new level of careful consideration.

Environmentally (i.e. under different scientific conditions), it is also important to show how autism plays out in different cultural contexts. In alignment with enactive theory, Ken Wilber's Integral Theory (Wilber, 1997) tries to show that growth and change of both an individual and an organisation is in constant interplay with the environment and other studies draw on the notion of epistemic communities to explore shifts in knowledge about autism, including concepts such as neurodiversity, and how these travel through cultural spaces. (O'Dell et al., 2016).

REFERENCES

Dawson, M. (2018). [Tweet, 10 August.] www.twitter.com/autismcrisis

Fletcher-Watson, S., et al. (2018). Making the future together: Shaping autism research through meaningful participation. Autism, 23(4). https://doi.org/10.1177/1362361318786721

O'Dell, L., Bertilsdotter Rosqvist, H., Ortega, F., Brownlow, C., & Orsini, M. (2016). Critical autism studies: exploring epistemic dialogues and intersections, challenging dominant understandings of autism. *Disability & Society*, 31(2), 166–179.

Wilber, K. (1997). An integral theory of consciousness. *Journal of Consciousness Studies*, 4(1), 71–92.

APPENDIX 7

An open letter about communication

....

This open letter addresses the inquest into the death of the author's brother, Paul Drury, questioning the role of Risperidone in his death. It highlights systemic failures in mental health care, communication issues, and the lack of attention to Paul's possible autism. The letter requests a review of the autopsy report to consider Risperidone's role.

IN MEMORY OF PAUL CHRISTOPHER MATTHEW DRURY

To: C.P. Dorries OBE
Office of H.M. Coroner
The Medico-Legal Centre,
Watery Street,
Sheffield, S3 7ES

Sheffield, UK
12th March 2018

Dear Mr Dorries,

Thank you for your letter dated 1st Feb 2018 regarding the inquest into my brother's death on 12th March 2006 and for your detailed considerations, given the time that has passed. I also thank you for providing copies of letters and the comprehensive report from Sheffield Care Trust, something that they refused me a viewing of 'due to the Limitation Act 1980' (their letter 8.1.18).

Today is the 12th anniversary of Paul's death. I chose to write this letter to you today for myself and it seems apt that twelve years is the maximum limit set by the government for a legal enquiry into assumed negligence.

Paul is 18 months younger than me and we grew up together. Last June 26th, which would've been his 50th birthday, I chose to open the autopsy report. I've always had a lingering question around his death. Your letter has clarified matters regarding the question about Risperidone being a contributory factor: 'On my understanding the Risperidone would not increase the quantity of alcohol found in your brother's body but it might have been the case that respiratory depression from the large quantity of alcohol would have been worsened.'

This view matches exactly the basis of my own enquiry and confirms exactly what I suspected and why I had a sense of something unresolved. I asked the Sheffield Care Trust, particularly Dr Fernandez (Michael Carlisle Centre) and Ian Shaw (Argyll House) what precautions were taken in the light of the known dangers of prescribing Risperidone for an alcoholic after seeing information on a public website: 'Severe Potential Hazard, High Plausibility. Applies to: Alcoholism. Severe respiratory depression and respiratory arrest may occur. Therapy with neuroleptic agents should be administered cautiously in patients who might be prone to acute alcohol intake.' (Drugs.com, n.d.)

In the public records I obtained, a letter to Fulwood House from Dr M. Fernandez points out that in November 2005, 'It was encouraging to see that Paul could cope with the discipline of a detoxification programme.' The 2006 report (by Roger Marshall, Mental Health Social Worker) which you also kindly provided reflects a change in Paul's behaviour after being prescribed Risperidone by Dr Fernandez in 2005, especially from December 2005, when this was altered to administration by injection:

'On 8th February 2006 Ian Shaw (Community Mental Health Nurse) visited Paul. Ian noted Paul's thought appeared less structured with incoherent speech – muttering to himself and unable to stay on the subject of discussion ... Ian administered Paul's depot injection as prescribed ... Paul claimed to be drinking two bottles of sherry per day.'

And 'On 10th March 2006 Paul was sitting outside Argyll House when Ian Shaw (Community Mental Health Nurse) arrived at work. Paul was drinking sherry and smoking a roll-up cigarette ...' 'Ian ... gave Paul his depot injection as prescribed.'

Paul died two days later.

Risperidone given to Paul, while highly intoxicated with alcohol, led to the 'severe respiratory depression and respiratory arrest' which you stated.

This should've been listed as (in the least) a contributory factor on the autopsy report (along with 1a. Ethanol poisoning. 2. Methadone use), should it not? Will you take into consideration these details and adjust the report accordingly? Your letter also states that because the amount of alcohol found in Paul's blood was '... well above the amount that would normally be regarded as the cause of death. It may therefore be that the pathologist would have regarded the Risperidone as irrelevant in those circumstances.'

It is very surprising to discover that your pathologist – upon reading the police report mentioning Paul's state – and the injection of Risperidone the day before he died (along with assumed general knowledge of the dangerous combinations) – did not carry out the standard test for it, deeming it 'irrelevant'. This gives me cause for concern.

In comparing atypical psychosis and autism, we find they frequently co-occur and both are linked to pronounced personality changes. Shared outcomes are difficulties in understanding others and loneliness, with stigma and discrimination likely exacerbating these and contributing towards experienced distress (Beattie, 2017).

There is a history of both autism and alcoholism in Paul's family. But there is no suggestion of suspected autism in any of the reports obtained. One of the three uses for Risperidone is named as 'irritability from autism'. I assume a neurological link to psychosis had already been made about Paul, but autism was never reportedly suspected by anyone in the large group of 'experts' who surrounded him. This I find odd. Can you see how poor the health system is in communicating with itself and the people it serves? There are massive failings inherent in our mental health systems and society, unfortunately driven largely by drug profiteers and the peddled myths in scientific cures. Whilst I accept the intense pathological views of autism is strong in society, introducing a chemical into the brain of an autistic person to somehow suppress irritability is at best questionable. Maybe we can assume autism wasn't ever checked. That would be even odder. It is shocking how little communication takes place across our communities with regards to autism and neurodiversity. Society has become so ridiculously infatuated by drugs and cures. The words 'care' and 'trust' in the Sheffield institution's name hold a dark irony yet it would be too convenient to attribute blame, I am only interested in facts.

Paul walked the streets for enjoyment, many people knew him. But he was shunted around services with multiple faces and viewpoints to contend with, and multiple dangerous drugs to try, administered by people basically working with the suppliers of all types. Signs were ignored and clinicians simply don't know what to do when, for example, as it's reported in the case notes, Paul was observed

- always avoiding talking about his family history
- his behaviour improving when a friend stayed with him
- his thinking and speech becoming more incoherent when starting a course of Risperidone
- stating he didn't want to take Risperidone.

Paul was someone clearly troubled in some social domains. The last time we spoke he told me he was going into rehab. But there was nothing 'wrong' with him. He was a fabulous, unusual, clever, unique and lovable guy and we, those who love him, celebrate his life.

And it seemed we had the last laugh together, as to this day I'm not entirely sure if we put him in the ground the right way round, which is bloody hilarious.

Kind regards,

Jonathan Drury
Dialogica UK

REFERENCES

Beattie, L. (2017). Autism and psychosis: what may be the role of social interactions? Retrieved from www.autscape.org/2017/programme/presentations

Drugs.com (n.d.). Risperidone disease interactions. Retrieved from www.drugs.com/disease-interactions/risperidone.html

Index

A

ableism 14, 56
Academy of Professional Dialogue 99, 104
ADHD 14, 71, 76, 126
Adler, Mortimer J. 122
Advaita Vedanta 16
alexithymia 86, 126
Aristotle 61–62, 65
Aron, Elaine 13
Asperger, Hans 7, 15
Atma Vichara 15
atopos 60
Augmented/assistive and Alternative Communication 86
authentic voice 41
autism: bringing together with dialogue 3–4, 28–35, 56–57, *see also* Autism Dialogue Approach; communication styles 53; definition of 48–49; discovery journey 13–18; existence and 124–125; peer-to-peer information transfer 53; theories and common themes 47–56; through social sciences lens 59–69; as way of being 49–50
Autism Dialogue Approach 3–4; aims of 39–40; beginnings of 5–8; benefits of 45; case examples 143–147, 148–152, 153–154, 155–159, 160–162; definition of 148–149; early sessions 32–35; facilitation skills 96–105; four practices 41–43, 100, 116, 117; hosting 85–94; Insight Dialogue and 116–118; mindfulness and 76–83; sensitive conversation 43–45; spirituality in 134–138; in therapy and coaching 123–131; training for facilitators 101; as transformative practice 131
Autism Dialogue Friends 153–154
Autism Industrial Complex 59
autistic culture 18–19

B

Bakhtin, Mikhail 34–35, 120
Ball, Jessica 42
Beardon, Luke 15
Belmonte, Matthew 60
Blejerman, Helen 8
Bleuler, Eugene 48–49
Bogdashina, Olga 32, 136–137
Bohm, David 5, 7, 19, 20–21, 29, 30, 31, 34, 39, 41, 43, 63, 64–65, 66, 68, 74, 77, 105, 113–114, 119–120, 134, 137
boundaries 93–94
British Association for Counsellors and Psychotherapists 99
Brown, Juanita 122
Buber, Martin 120–121
Buddhism 9, 24, 62–63, 77, 80, 117
bullying 56

C

change, resistance to 140–142
Chown, Nick 10, 32, 59–60
Christianity 80

Circles of Trust 121
closure 94
cognitive behavioural therapies 127
communication breakdown 68–69
communication styles 53; non-violent communication 135; open letter regarding 166–168
Confucianism 24, 62
contracting 88–90
COVID-19 pandemic 67–68, 98, 148
creativity 100
Crenshaw, Kimberlé 109–110
Crompton, Catherine J. 53
Cycle of Liberation 113–114
Cycle of Socialisation 113–114

D

Dalai Lama 7, 63, 134
David Bohm Society 134
De Jaegher, Hanne 61, 63–64
Derby Clinical Commissioning Group 143–144
Descartes, René 61, 64, 67
Di Paolo, Ezequiel 126
dialogic supervision 129
Dialogue: bringing together with autism 3–4, 28–35, 56–57, *see also* Autism Dialogue Approach; and communication breakdown 68–69; definition of 20–21; East and West 24–25; in indigenous societies 22–24; Insight Dialogue 80, 116–118, 119; intergroup 111–114; intersectionality and 109–114; in practice 25–27; professional 104–105; as a system 62–63; through social sciences lens 59–69; in traditional communities/societies 21–22
digital spaces 60, 68, 97–98
double empathy problem 52, 125, 135, 140
Dunbar, Robin 21
Dyer, Wayne 78

E

echolalia 74, 82, 86
effortless effort 81–82
Eliot, T. S. 82
enactive approach 63, 68, 125–128
ethics 93, 98–99
eugenics 7
European Mentoring and Coaching Council 99
Evolutionary-Stress Framework 22
executive dysfunction 50
existence 124–125
Explicate Order 64–65

F

facilitation skills 96–105
feedback 94
Foucault, Michel 137
four practices 41–43, 100, 116, 117; authentic voice 41; listening 41–42, 104, 157; respect 42; suspension 42
Freire, Paulo 4, 118–119

G

Garrett, Peter 10
gestalt coaching 123–124, 156
gestalt processing 73–75
Grandin, Temple 137

H

Hallaq, W. 137
Harris, Paul 49
Harro, Bobbie 113
Higham, Nic 15, 129
highly sensitive people 13–14, 52
Hinduism 9, 24
Hodge, Nick 31, 60
Hogenkamp, Lori 6, 22, 51–52
hyper-empathy 15
hypersensitivity 59

I

Ibn Arabi 137
Implicate Order *see* Theory of the Implicate Order
indigenous societies 22–24
Insight Dialogue 80, 116–118, 119
intellectual disability 50
Intense World Theory of Autism 54
Intergroup Dialogue 111–114
interoception 81
interpretative phenomenological analysis 100
intersectionality 109–114
Isaacs, David 122
Isaacs, William 4, 20, 39, 41
Islam 80

K

Kanner, Leo 49
koinonia 34, 96
Kramer, Gregory 116–117
Krishnamurti, J. 7, 134

L

leadership culture 141–142
learning disability 50

Leigh-Holt, Allison 28–29
listening 41–42, 104, 157
lockdown 67–68, 98, 148
loneliness 56
Long, Katherine 155

M

Manning, Erin 6, 29–30, 72, 74, 80
mantras 82–83
Markram, Henry and Kamila 54
masking 16–17, 30, 54–55, 128–129
Maturana, Humberto 62–63
Milne, Liz 5
Milton, Damian 6, 52, 60, 127
mindful awareness 31–32, 79–80
mindfulness 31–32, 66, 76–83, 117, 136
Mindfulness for Autism 76
Miserandino, Christine 136
monotropism 50–51, 54
Murray, Dinah 39

N

National Autistic Society 97
nature of self 61–62
neurodiversity 71–75; and autistic gestalt processing 73–74; need for 74–75; problems with 72–73
New Economics Foundation 79
Newton, Isaac 65, 67
Nondual Therapy 129
Non-Violent Communication 119, 135

O

organisations, working with 102–104

P

Palmer, Parker J. 121
paradigm shift in therapy 130–131
participatory research 163–164
Participatory Sense-Making 126–127
Pedagogy of the Oppressed 118–119
peer-to-peer information transfer 53
'peripheral minds' framework 6
Personal Wellness Index 8
phenomenology 63, 67, 163–164
Piaget, Jean 49
Plato 61
predominant neurotype 49–50, 57, 64
professional dialogue 104–105
PTSD 18, 86, 123

Q

Quakers 121

R

race 109–110, 112, 126
Reeve, Hester 8, 65
relational humility 130–131
respect 42
responsibility 98–99
rituals 136
Rosenberg, Marshall 135

S

safe spaces 129–130
self, nature of 61–62
self-acceptance 80–81
self-harm 47, 56, 60, 67, 81, 93
self-organising principle 66
sensitive conversation 43–45
sensory sensitivity 54
Siegel, Daniel 125
Silberman, Steve 7
silence 5, 78–79, 92, 125, 161
Singer, Judy 71
Smith, Richard 5
social anxiety 118, 143, 149, 158
Socratic Seminar 119, 121–122
spiritual interaction 119–121
spirituality 93, 134–138
Stillman, William 137
stimming 88; vocal 86
Stress Adaptation theory 6, 51–52
Sufism 9, 19, 24, 62, 137
suicide/ideation 47, 56, 59–60, 67, 81, 88, 93
suspension 42
systemic trauma 65–67

T

talking 124
Tao 9, 19, 24, 62
Theory of Mind 50, 64
Theory of the Implicate Order 7, 29, 30, 64–65, 68–69
traditional communities/societies 21–22
trauma 14, 55–56, 60, 76, 127; systemic 65–67
triggers 88

U

uncertainty 99–100
Uribe, Rodrigo 62–63

V

Varela, Francisco 62–63
vocal stimming 86

W

Wagener, Helena 102
weak central coherence 50
Wholeness and the Implicate
 Order *see* Theory of the Implicate Order
Williams, Donna 137
World Café 119, 122

Y

Yalom, Irvin 128

Z

Zen 9, 19, 33
Zoom 98, 148

For Product Safety Concerns and Information please contact our
EU representative GPSR@taylorandfrancis.com Taylor & Francis
Verlag GmbH, Kaufingerstraße 24, 80331 München, Germany